When God's People Have
HIV/AIDS

When God's People Have HIV/AIDS

An Approach to Ethics

MARIA CIMPERMAN, OSU

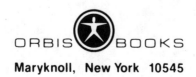
ORBIS BOOKS
Maryknoll, New York 10545

Founded in 1970, Orbis Books endeavors to publish works that enlighten the mind, nourish the spirit, and challenge the conscience. The publishing arm of the Maryknoll Fathers and Brothers, Orbis seeks to explore the global dimensions of the Christian faith and mission, to invite dialogue with diverse cultures and religious traditions, and to serve the cause of reconciliation and peace. The books published reflect the views of their authors and do not represent the official position of the Maryknoll Society. To learn more about Maryknoll and Orbis Books, please visit our website at www.maryknoll.org.

Copyright © 2005 by Maria Cimperman.

Published by Orbis Books, Maryknoll, New York 10545-0308.

Manufactured in the United States of America.

Queries regarding rights and permissions should be addressed to: Orbis Books, P.O. Box 308, Maryknoll, New York 10545-0308.

Library of Congress Cataloging-in-Publication Data

Cimperman, Maria.
  When God's people have HIV/AIDS: an approach to ethics / Maria Cimperman.
      p. cm.
  Includes bibliographical references and index.
  ISBN-13: 978-1-57075-623-8 (pbk.)
  1. AIDS (Disease)—Religious aspects—Catholic Church. 2. Christian ethics—Catholic authors. I. Title.
  BX2347.8.A52C56 2005
  261.8′321969792—dc22
                  2005009303

To all persons infected or affected by HIV/AIDS

To those whose ministry is prevention or treatment and care of persons
at risk of or infected with HIV/AIDS

To all who struggle to eradicate HIV/AIDS through the elimination
of poverty and gender inequality

Contents

Acknowledgments

*I thank my God every time I remember you, constantly praying with joy in
every one of my prayers for all of you.*

(Phil. 1:3–4)

I must admit to being shaped and formed by many persons, narratives, and
cultures along the way to the publication of this book. It began as a dissertation, and it is abundantly clear to me that one cannot write a dissertation or
a book without a community. And it is to more than one community that I
offer my deep gratitude. I begin with my family. My mom, dad, and brother,
from childhood on, in many ways called me to probe with depth both my faith
and the needs of the world around me. I especially thank my brother, Joe,
for his love and friendship and his example to me of what an option for the
poor, vulnerable, and marginalized looks like among the people of God today.
For being a wonderful conversation and dialogue partner on the topics that
really matter, I thank you!

I am very grateful to my congregation, the Ursuline Sisters of Cleveland.
They continue to offer encouragement and support with prayer and friendship. Dorothy Kazel, OSU, martyred in El Salvador in 1980 with and among
the people of God, has been a key inspiration for my studies and work in areas
of justice. Special thanks too to Maureen McCarthy, OSU, who was general
superior of our congregation when she encouraged the start of graduate studies and offered her blessings in countless ways over the years. And I continue
to be grateful for our congregational direction statements, which call and challenge us to transformation based on contemplation, justice, and compassion
and to focus our ministries on empowerment, direct service, and systemic
change for and among the oppressed, especially women and children, both
locally and globally.

I have had the blessing of living and ministering with a variety of congre-
gations during my studies. So I offer warm thanks to the Religious of the
Sacred Heart of Jesus and the Mercy Sisters of Providence, all of whom in
various ways offered hospitality, community, and inspiration for engaging

theological ethics. I also thank my colleagues from the Cardinal Suenens Center conference on The Nun in the Postmodern World. They taught me much about collegiality and scholarship and helped me hear the call to grow more fully and more deeply as both a woman religious and a theologian. Finally, thanks to the Columban community, which offered me hospitality during the summer the writing was completed, and to the Sisters of the Incarnate Word in San Antonio, who welcomed me as the editing drew to a close.

Today I particularly thank my colleagues and the students at the Oblate School of Theology, who encouraged the publication of a work on AIDS. Special thanks too to Susan Perry, Catherine Costello, and the staff of Orbis Books, whose Gospel commitment to the needs of the poor and marginalized support works such as this, so that more ways may be found to respond to the cries of the people of God.

I am deeply grateful for the blessing of incredible mentors on my journey toward becoming a theologian. Jim Keenan, SJ, not only directed the thesis on which this book is based, but also helped deepen and widen my vision. His passionate teaching and engagement at all levels and among all people have provided an inspiring image of the theologian as a person of faith, a scholar, and an activist. Jim helped me find my own voice and encouraged me to trust its truth—for this I owe a great debt of gratitude. Lisa Sowle Cahill's breadth of knowledge and abiding concern for the common good and those on the margins brought an essential lens to this project. Jon Fuller, SJ, MD, has been a wonderful resource and inspiration through both his clinical work and policy insights. His theological insights were helpful as this project addressed the intersections of medicine and theology. His keen eye for detail continues to teach me a great deal.

My Boston College and Weston Jesuit School of Theology communities have been great places of grace-filled opportunities for growth and friendship. I learned much from working with James Weiss and Michael Himes. The Boston College Ignatio Volunteer program staff and participants kept me grounded and challenged me to put flesh on the theology and ethics I was engaging.

I am very grateful for mentors in my life over these years of graduate study and growth. Thanks to Maura Ryan at the University of Notre Dame for encouraging me to pursue further work in theological ethics and for her ongoing wisdom. I particularly wish to thank three wisdom women in my life—Judith Anne Beattie, CSC; Meg Guider, OSF; and Dorothy Cotterell, SUSC—who mentored me in both holiness and wholeness.

Friends are one of life's greatest blessings, and I thank God for these incarnations of love in my life. I particularly want to mention Ursuline friends Janet Moore, Joanne Gross, and Anita Whitely. Janet, thank you for your friendship throughout my Ursuline journey. And Joanne, thank you also for your time and talent in kindly editing the dissertation as the writing came to a close.

January 27, 2005
Feast of St. Angela Merici

The Genesis of a Book

AIDS

Should anyone ask you the reason for this hope of y
reply, but speak gently and respectfully.

—

When I first began researching and writing on HIV/A
asked why I was writing on this topic. I had just spent a
West Africa, and some wondered whether my interest w
Many presumed that I had had some kind of personal expe
AIDS. Some wondered what would compel me to write on a
rife with political and theological landmines. People consistentl
AIDS?" and most wanted a personal response rather than an ac

At first, I found the question perplexing: "Why write about A
disease is a global pandemic. Do I need a personal reason other tha
a human being and there are millions of human beings around
dying of AIDS? Is not AIDS a global issue of concern to all? In time, hov.
I realized that we set out in certain directions because we find ourselves co.
nected somehow to a person, a topic, a people. The heart, the head, and the
entire being become involved, and the more we share that involvement, the
more we invite others into the world around us.

Why do I, as a theologian, write about AIDS? Because theology and praxis
cannot be separated from the reality of a world with AIDS. Because although
theology and ethics are timeless, their application is shaped in each age by
people living in a dynamic world. Most importantly, I write because the people of God live with HIV/AIDS. And theology and ethics must be lived and
practiced in the midst of the people of God.

I first learned about the stigma and isolation of AIDS from my brother
Joe. In the early 1990s, he was a Jesuit Volunteer Corps (JVC) member in a
Baltimore AIDS hospice, predominantly ministering to gay men. I had the
opportunity to visit him at this ministry, to meet some of the men, and to
hear their stories. About a week after my visit, Joe called me one morning.

lift during which John[1], one of the resi-
could do was hold him and tell him that
his shift that morning, John told Joe that he
him and touched him gently and reverently

He had just returned from a
dents, sobbed and sobbed
he was loved. As my br
was the first person   ent eight weeks in Ghana, West Africa, studying
since his diagnosi   and medicine as it affected healing in a cross-
In the summe   w the face of AIDS and its ominous potential in
the intersect   a.   apacity to prevent the AIDS devastation that had

cultural c   many billboards on the major highways advertising
a count   the young people I spoke with knew about AIDS and
hit o   African regions that were suffering from AIDS. However,
rn region and town of Tamale, none of the sexually active
met used a condom. A general comment I heard from them
did not have the virus, so they could not transmit the virus dur-
tivity. Some considered HIV infection to be random and likened
the guinea worm in a pool of water. Why, they asked, is it that
e can drink from the same water source, yet one gets guinea worm
other not? Perhaps, they suggested, it is simply a matter of fate.

se conversations alarmed me because I knew both that the virus was
dy present and that its spread could be curbed. Ghana, especially this
on of the country, was still in the early stages of the spread of the virus.
t there were signs that this would not be so for long. Local health workers
stimated that about 80% of the sex workers in Tamale were HIV-positive.
These sex workers often began their careers as early as their pre-teen years,
working for basics such as food and clothing.[2] Their customers were mostly
farmers who regularly came to the market in town to buy and trade goods.
These farmers would remain in town for three or four days before returning to their villages and families.

Most female sex workers did not ask their partners to use a prophylactic. Condoms were not yet culturally acceptable, and many men did not
find their sexual experience as pleasurable when they used a condom.[3]

A week before I left the region, a woman with end-stage AIDS came to
the Shekinah Clinic, where I had been volunteering and interviewing patients
and staff. Because I had heard that Cecilia was near death, I did not want to
intrude on this sacred care-giving time for her and for the staff. However,
the staff asked her to share her story with me. They believed it important that
I meet this person and hear a story that they were hearing with increasing fre-
quency. They wanted to help me understand what was happening in their
land and among their people. Cecilia consented, and the next day, lying on
a mat on the floor, barely able to lift her head, she shared her story.

Cecilia was the mother of four children, the two youngest of whom had
already died of AIDS, or "slim disease," as it is also called. Her husband,
Moses, had died of the disease three years earlier. Moses had traveled every

month to Tamale to trade, and he was often gone three or four days at a time. Moses was the first in the village to have slim disease, though many had heard of other traders getting the disease. While Cecilia took care of Moses during his illness, the family lived in the husband's village, but after he died, Moses's family asked her to leave and to take the children. The two younger children were now also sickly, and Moses's relatives were afraid that the disease would spread to them. Cecilia moved back to her family's village and was able to care for her two youngest children until they died. By then her own physical condition had worsened, so she asked her sisters to care for the two older children. Not wanting her remaining children to see yet another family member die, Cecilia left them. She died four days after arriving at the Shekinah Clinic.

The spring after returning from Ghana, I took an "AIDS and Casuistry" course with moral theologian James Keenan, SJ, and physician Jon Fuller, SJ. The other people taking the course were from around the world and from a variety of disciplines—theology, law, medicine, social work, and education. I quickly learned that a global consideration of HIV/AIDS is essential for both prevention and treatment efforts. It was during this semester that I began to realize that HIV/AIDS was a disease that would truly change the course not only of global health care, politics, economics, and law, but also theology. The AIDS crisis is calling us all to look more deeply at our moral theology if we are to respond to the "signs of the times" and offer hope.

And lest one think that HIV affects only the poor, minorities, or persons beyond our borders, I would like to share a narrative of a woman living in Cleveland, Ohio. In the process of interviewing experts on the domestic and global dimensions of HIV/AIDS, I met Earl Pike, executive director of the AIDS Task Force of Greater Cleveland. His introduction to me was by way of sharing the conversation he had had just moments before I walked into his office. A Caucasian woman living in a higher income suburb had called with some questions. She began, however, by stating that there were two things Earl needed to know and understand before she asked anything. First, she is a Christian, and her church does not believe in divorce. Second, her religion requires a wife to be submissive to her husband. The woman then proceeded to describe lesions on her husband's back. She also shared that she had found porn magazines in his closet that morning while she was cleaning. Earl asked a series of questions. Can you talk to your husband about the lesions? No. Can you ask your husband to go to the doctor? No. Can you ask your husband to use a condom or to refrain from sexual intercourse? No. Can you refuse sex with your husband? No. Finally, Earl had no more questions and there was a long pause. The woman finally broke the silence: "Am I going to die of AIDS, too?" Clearly, the influence of religion cannot be ignored.

In the summer of 2002, I accompanied Boston College undergraduates to Jamaica for a three-week service and immersion and theological reflection experience. In the hills of rural Jamaica, I was asked to pray with a young woman who was sick. Jennie was twenty-three years old and had returned the previous week from six weeks in a nearby hospital. Her extended family had spent their entire savings on her stay there. She received no diagnosis, but was sent home with antidiarrhea medicine and vitamins. She was dying of AIDS, but no one diagnosed her or told her family. The doctors and nurses in the Jamaican hospital did not use the words "HIV-positive" or "AIDS," even though they were treating Jennie and numerous others with similarly emaciated bodies and other common symptoms.

More recently my conversion experiences have included participation in the San Antonio ACTS (Adoration, Community, Theology, Service) retreat and follow-up for persons infected with or affected by HIV/AIDS. In addition to persons infected with HIV/AIDS, the participants include family members who have lost a loved one to the disease and social workers, health-care workers, and others who minister to the HIV community. At these gatherings I heard not only the violent voice of HIV, but also the equally powerful lived responses of persons with the disease. While sharing the challenges of living with a virus that threatens his life, Sergio succinctly articulated his response to HIV: "This is not my time to die. It is my time to live."

A convergence of these and other experiences and a great deal of information and insight gained from Jim Keenan and Jon Fuller continue to drive my work on foundational ethics in light of the AIDS pandemic. The global and local needs are immediate and pressing. And the Catholic tradition contains rich resources that can address not only the immediate concerns of HIV/AIDS prevention and treatment, but also the long-term problems that contribute to the pandemic.

In the preface to the *Report on the Global HIV/AIDS Epidemic, 2002,* Peter Piot, executive director of the Joint United Nations Program on HIV/AIDS, wrote: "In 2001, the world marked 20 years of AIDS. It was an occasion to lament the fact that the epidemic has turned out to be far worse than predicted, saying, *'if we knew then what we know now'.* But we do know now. We know the epidemic is still in its early stages, that effective responses are possible but only when they are politically backed and full-scale, and that unless more is done today and tomorrow, the epidemic will continue to grow."[4] What began as a serious health crisis in the early 1990s has now become a pandemic that affects the very foundations of society.[5] Not only is HIV/AIDS affecting the global physical health of persons; it is also ravaging the social, economic, and political well-being of peoples and nations.

The Second Vatican Council document, *Gaudium et Spes,* sagely exhorts us to "read the signs of the times" and to respond to them with our available resources.[6] "The total number of people living with the human immunodeficiency virus (HIV) rose in 2004 to reach its highest level ever: an estimated 39.4 million [35.9 million–44.3 million] people are living with the virus . . . This figure includes the 4.9 million [4.3 million–6.4 million] people who acquired HIV in 2004. The global AIDS epidemic killed 3.1 million

[2.8 million–3.5 million] people in the past year."[7] These are alarming signs of our times.

This book is a constructive proposal for fundamental ethics within the global context of HIV/AIDS. To bring our resources to bear on the AIDS pandemic, we must first understand these "signs of the times." The first chapter offers a brief look at the indicators of the AIDS pandemic and includes a discussion of two foundational contributors of the pandemic: gender inequality and poverty. The resources the Roman Catholic tradition and community bring to the HIV/AIDS crisis and some of the challenges with which the tradition is contending are explored. The final section of the chapter poses the question that serves as the focus of this project, namely, What kind of moral theology do we need in a world with AIDS? As a contribution to ongoing efforts in moral theology, this book explores the type of theological anthropology needed in a time of AIDS.

Chapters 2 and 3 develop a theological anthropology that considers human beings as embodied relational agents. The context explored here is one marked by great historical suffering. The agent described must develop or cultivate particular qualities, and the virtues name those qualities.

Chapter 4 examines how the virtues fill out our anthropological framework. Specific virtues that respond to particular elements of the HIV/AIDS crisis are highlighted, including hope, fidelity, self-care, justice, and prudence.

The final three chapters seek to animate the embodied, virtue-oriented anthropology of the preceding chapters. An integrated sense of spirituality and morality within the context of discipleship is necessary for the church community to propose an anthropology to adequately respond to HIV/AIDS. This idea is developed in three parts. In Chapter 5, Christian spirituality and Christian morality are defined and discussed within the context of discipleship. In Chapter 6, memory, narrative, and solidarity are explored. In Chapter 7, two contemporary examples of discipleship in this age of AIDS are considered: Noerine Kaleeba of Uganda and Paul Farmer of the United States.

God's people have HIV/AIDS, and our calling as disciples is to bring our theological and human resources to the service of God's people. Let us begin.

CHAPTER 1

Constructing a Fundamental Ethics
for an Age of HIV/AIDS

*The Church has always had the duty of scrutinizing the signs of the times
and of interpreting them in the light of the gospel.*
Vatican Council II, *Gaudium et Spes*, no. 4

In order to bring our resources to bear on the AIDS pandemic, let us first understand some of these "signs of the times." We begin with a brief look at the indicators of the pandemic: the methods of transmission, the demographics of the pandemic, and current prevention and treatment strategies for HIV/AIDS.

INDICATORS OF THE PANDEMIC[1]

Modes of Transmission

The human immunodeficiency virus (HIV) causes the acquired immune deficiency syndrome (AIDS). The National Institute of Allergy and Infectious Diseases (NIAID) explains: "By killing or impairing cells of the immune system, HIV progressively destroys the body's ability to fight infections and certain cancers. Individuals diagnosed with AIDS are susceptible to life-threatening diseases called opportunistic infections, which are caused by microbes that usually do not cause illness in healthy people."[2]

HIV can be transmitted in a number of ways. The most common method of transmission is through sex with an infected partner. The virus can enter the body "through the lining of the vagina, vulva, penis, rectum or mouth during sex."[3] HIV is also frequently spread among injecting drug users through the sharing of needles or syringes contaminated with minuscule amounts of blood from a person infected with the virus. Similarly, while screening of blood in industrialized countries has greatly reduced the incidence of infection,

HIV can be spread through transfusion of contaminated blood or blood components.[4] Women can also transmit HIV to their children during pregnancy or birth or through breast milk.[5] According to UNAIDS/WHO, "Fewer than 10% of pregnant women are currently offered services of proven effectiveness to prevent HIV transmission during pregnancy and childbirth."[6]

Changing Demographics

As of the end of 2002, an estimated 36.6 million adults and children were estimated to be living with HIV. By the end of 2004, the numbers increased to 39.4 million persons living with HIV. A regional breakdown of the numbers of adults and children estimated to be living with HIV/AIDS at the end of 2002 and 2004 is given in Table 1.[7]

Table 1. Number of Adults and Children Living with HIV, by Region

Region	End of 2002	End of 2004[8]
Oceania	28,000 [22,000–38,000]	35,000 [25,000–48,000]
Caribbean	420,000 [260,000–740,000]	440,000 [270,000–780,000]
N. Africa & Middle East	430,000 [180,000–1.2 million]	540,000 [230,000–1.5 million]
Western and Central Europe	600,000 [470,000–750,000]	610,000 [480,000–760,000]
East Asia	760,000 [380,000–1.2 million]	1.1 million [560,000–1.8 million]
North America	970,000 [500,000–1.6 million]	1 million [540,000–1.6 million]
Eastern Europe & Central Asia	1 million [670,000–1.5 million]	1.4 million [920,000–2.1 million]
Latin America	1.5 million [1.1–2 million]	1.7 million [1.3–2.2 million]
South and Southeast Asia	6.4 million [3.9–9.7 million]	7.1 million [4.4–10.6 million]
Sub-Saharan Africa	24.4 million [22.5–27.3 million]	25.4 million [23.4–28.4 million]
Total	36.6 million	39.4 million

Let us briefly look a bit more closely at some of the regions and countries whose numbers of HIV+ incidence continue to increase. Since June 1981, when the HIV/AIDS epidemic was first reported in the United States, demographics have shifted significantly. In the early years, AIDS in the United States was considered to primarily affect gay white males, but now new populations are being infected, and increasing numbers of people are being infected through unprotected heterosexual intercourse.[9] Newly diagnosed AIDS cases from heterosexual transmission have risen "from 3% in 1985 to 31% in 2003. Over that same period, the share of new AIDS diagnoses due to sex between men fell from 65% to 42%. The share of AIDS diagnoses due to injection drug use was 19% in 1985, peaking at 31% in 1993, and was 22% in 2003."[10]

Increasing numbers of infections are coming from members of minority communities.[11] The epidemic "is now disproportionately lodged among African Americans and is affecting much greater numbers of women."[12] Studies have revealed that: "Although African Americans represent just 12% of the country's population, over half of new HIV diagnoses in recent years have been among them . . . Especially affected are African American women, who account for up to 72% of new HIV diagnoses in all US women. At the turn of the century already, AIDS ranked among the top three causes of death for African American men aged 25–54 and for African American women aged 35–44 years."[13] Latinos (male and female) account for 20% of new cases, even though they are only 14% of the U.S. population.[14] Latinas account for 16% of new AIDS diagnoses among women in 2003.[15] Among women in general, heterosexual intercourse "accounts for most HIV diagnoses among women, and there are strong indications that the main risk factor for many women acquiring HIV is the often-undisclosed risk behaviour of their male partners."[16]

Data show that HIV/AIDS is continuing to move into "poorer and more marginalized sections of society."[17] The UNAIDS Report states that "It should go without saying that race and ethnicity are not per se risk factors for HIV. Poverty and other forms of socioeconomic deprivation, however, are known to increase vulnerability to HIV infection."[18] Nearly one in four African Americans and one in five Hispanics live in poverty.[19] Some U.S. studies indicate a "close relationship between higher AIDS incidence and lower income."[20] Finally, although AIDS-related deaths have declined since the introduction of antiretroviral therapy in 1995–1996, "the rate of death due to AIDS among African Americans was over twice as high as that among whites in 2002. African Americans now have the poorest survival rates among people diagnosed with AIDS—probably reflecting late diagnoses (often after the disease has become symptomatic) and inadequate access to quality health care services."[21]

The worst affected region in the world is sub-Saharan Africa, with 25.4 million people living with HIV. With only 10% of the global population, the region is home to over 60% of all persons living with HIV. In 2004 an estimated 3.1 million adults and children became newly infected, and the AIDS epidemic claimed the lives of an estimated 2.3 million persons in the past year.[22] "Among young people aged 15–24 years, an estimated 6.9% [6.3–8.3%] of women and 2.2% [2.0–2.7%] of men were living with HIV at the end of 2004."[23] HIV+ prevalence rates of over 20% are estimated for six sub-Saharan countries. With an estimated 21.5% adult prevalence rate (5.3 million people), South Africa is home to the largest number of people living with HIV/AIDS in the world.[24] The highest prevalence rates in the world are in sub-Saharan Africa, with Swaziland ranked first (38.8%), followed by Botswana (37.3%).[25]

The challenges in Africa are enormous. In southern Africa, life expectancy at birth is now below 40 years in nine countries: Botswana, Central African Republic, Lesotho, Malawi, Mozambique, Rwanda, Swaziland, Zambia, and Zimbabwe.[26] There are an estimated 12 million children living in sub-Saharan Africa who are AIDS orphans (with one or more parents lost because of the pandemic).[27]

There are some signs of hope in the midst of these daunting figures. One positive trend is from East Africa and Uganda, where the "national prevalence fell from 13% in the early 1990s to 4.1% (2.8–6.6%) by end-2003."[28] Recent data suggest Kenya could be experiencing a similar decline, as "data from antenatal clinics show median HIV prevalence falling from 13.6% (12.2–27.1%) in 1997–1998 to 9.4% (6.6–14.3%) in 2002 and staying largely unchanged in 2003."[29] This suggests that awareness and prevention programs are helping. However, challenges persist, because even if new infections were to stop immediately, the human and socioeconomic effects will be felt for generations.

Although national prevalence rates in most countries in Asia are relatively low when compared with those in Africa (Cambodia, Myanmar, and Thailand are exceptions), this information can be misleading: "Within the largest Asian nations, some geographic regions have far more inhabitants than most African countries and have HIV prevalence rates far greater than the national average. In Asian countries in which the epidemic is concentrated in certain groups, such as injecting drug users, it is misleading to focus solely on the prevalence in the general population."[30] India and China are the two most populous nations in the world, with a combined 2.35 billion people. So a low prevalence rate in India, for example (the national adult HIV prevalence rate is less than 1%), still amounts to an estimated 5.1 million (2.5–5.8 million) persons living with HIV in 2003, second only to South Africa's figures.[31] It is assumed that China and India will be part of the epidemic's "next wave" if intervention efforts are not significantly increased and expanded over this decade.[32]

The numbers are significant: 1.2 million (720,000–2.4 million) people in Asia acquired HIV in 2004, bringing the number of people now living with the virus to an estimated 8.2 million (5.4–11.8 million). A further 540,000 (350,000–810,000) people in Asia are estimated to have died of AIDS in the past year.[33]

Significantly, the official Chinese news media have published a number of articles about China's growing AIDS problem, acknowledging not only an urban epidemic (in which HIV is believed to be transmitted primarily through sex workers and injecting drug users), but also a rural epidemic where transmission is occurring through the illegal sale of blood by poor farmers.[34] Although the HIV epidemic is diverse in terms of nature, pace, and severity across regions in China, much of the spread of HIV continues to be a result of injecting drug use and paid sex.[35] Studies are showing that "sexual transmission of HIV from injecting drug users to their sex partners looks certain to feature more prominently in China's fast-evolving epidemic."[36] A serious challenge is that "inadequate prevention efforts have allowed the virus to filter from people with the highest-risk behaviours (such as non-sterile drug injection and unprotected commercial sex) to their regular sex partners, which accounts for rising HIV-infection levels among women who report having only one sexual partner."[37]

Reports also indicate that "there are signs that efforts to boost public knowledge about HIV are bearing fruit, but there remains much room for improvement. A 2003 survey found that two-in-five Chinese men and women could not name a single way to protect themselves against infection."[38] In addition, there are concerns that "massive population mobility (an estimated 100 million Chinese are temporarily or permanently away from their registered addresses), and increasing socio-economic disparities add to the likelihood of wider HIV spread."[39] The UNAIDS/WHO *AIDS Epidemic Update: December 2004* states that China "can still shape the course of its epidemic. But it needs to move swiftly and with great resolve."[40]

Treatment for HIV is a topic that some countries are addressing. Although less than 6% of the 170,000 persons in need of antiretrovirals in Asia are receiving it, "Thailand appears on track to reach its target of providing 50,000 people with antiretroviral treatment, while others have committed themselves to drastically expand treatment access—including Cambodia, China (which has pledged free treatment in several states) and Indonesia."[41] This is a hopeful note in contrast to the 2002 warning from Nicholas Eberstadt, holder of the Henry Wendt Chair in Political Economy at the American Enterprise Institute and Senior Policy Adviser to the National Bureau of Asian Research, that even if treatment were free in Eurasian states, the cost of distributing the drugs would be more than the "economic value to governments of the lives saved."[42]

The 2002 UNAIDS/WHO *AIDS Epidemic Update* warned that the "epidemics in Latin America and the Caribbean are well established. There is a danger that they could spread both more quickly and more widely in the absence of strengthened responses."[43] Estimates made in 2004 show that in many areas this warning has come true. More than 2 million children and adults are estimated to be living with HIV in these regions—a figure that includes the estimated 290,000 people who acquired the virus in 2004. Five countries in the Caribbean have adult HIV prevalence rates exceeding 2%, making the Caribbean the second-most affected region in the world. AIDS is now the leading cause of death among adults aged 15–44 years in the region.[44] Haiti's adult prevalence rate is the worst, at 5.6%.[45] Yet in the midst of the challenges in these regions, there are signs that "the epidemic does yield to appropriate and resolute responses."[46]

Brazil is illustrative in terms of both the spread of the virus and treatment initiatives. The epidemic at first was mainly distributed among men who have sex with men and among injecting drug users. Now heterosexual transmission accounts for a growing number of HIV infections, and women are increasingly affected.[47] One study reports that "overall, 7% of the sex workers were HIV-positive, but among those living in urban slums, HIV levels were 18% and among illiterate women in their ranks they reached 23%."[48] The Brazilian government has an initiative to recruit and offer testing to all pregnant women, to provide treatment to prevent mother-to-child transmission, and to treat infected women and their infants.[49]

Other Latin American countries are also showing the increasing feminization of the epidemic and a decrease in the ratio of men with HIV infections to women with HIV infections. In Argentina, "throughout the 1980s and much of the 1990s, HIV transmission occurred mainly through injecting drug use, predominantly involving men. But sexual transmission of HIV—mainly from infected drug users to their female partners, as well as between men who have sex with men—has become more prominent, accounting for an estimated 80% of all reported AIDS cases . . . and the male-to-female ratio among people living with HIV narrowed from 15:1 in 1988 to 3:1 in 2002. Most new infections appear to be occurring among the poorest and least-educated urban inhabitants."[50] While in the Andean region HIV was primarily in the population of sex workers, their clients, and men who have sex with men, increasingly the virus is being spread to the wives and girlfriends of these men.[51] One study in Lima, Peru, found that "almost 90% of HIV-positive pregnant women had had just one or two sex partners in their lifetimes."[52] Another report affirmed that "the women's HIV risk depended almost exclusively on the sexual behaviour of their male partners, and those most at risk were young women."[53] In the Central American countries of Guatemala, Honduras, Nicaragua, Panama, and El Salvador, various ministries of health state that a large proportion of men who have sex with men also report having female sexual partners. Prevention efforts must address this information. "Bisexuality therefore constitutes a significant bridge for HIV transmission into the wider population. Similarly, the wives or regular partners of sex worker clients face an elevated risk of HIV infection, even when they themselves have only one sex partner."[54]

Also helping to drive the spread of HIV is "a combination of unequal socioeconomic development and high population mobility."[55] Central America's worsening epidemic is due to a population driven to itinerancy because of high unemployment and great poverty, concentrated mainly among socially marginalized populations.[56]

Another growing area of concern is the spread of HIV through sharing of needles used for injecting drugs. Brazil's very focused prevention programs for injecting drug users resulted in a substantial decrease in HIV prevalence among this population in several large metropolitan areas.[57] In terms of treatment, Brazil is a sign of hope among developing countries. All persons living with HIV have access to antiretroviral drugs through its national health system. As a result, survival rates of AIDS patients are increasing dramatically. Further good news is that in several countries, including Argentina, Costa Rica, and Panama, AIDS cases and AIDS mortality also declined after access to antiretroviral treatment was expanded.[58]

In the Caribbean, heterosexual intercourse is the primary mode of HIV transmission. More women are being infected as the epidemic evolves in this region, and new infections among women now exceed those among men.[59] Again, "poorer, less educated women are more likely to be HIV-infected than their better-off counterparts."[60] Guyana has the second highest prevalence rate in the region (2.5%) and has experienced a steep rise in HIV cases reported since the mid-1990s. However, according to the Ministry of Health, fewer than one-fifth of persons infected (the majority between the ages of 20 and 34 years) are aware of their HIV status.[61] A recent study showed an exceptionally high prevalence rate (6.5%) among mine workers in Guyana's Amazon region. The miners are all young men and divide their time, working for six to eight weeks in the mines and then going to their homes near the coast for two weeks.[62] There is a similar concern over the high prevalence rate (4.9%) among sugarcane plantation workers in the Dominican Republic.[63] Meanwhile, in Barbados, there has been a decline in HIV-infected pregnant women, and mother-to-child transmission has decreased by 69% since voluntary counseling and testing services were expanded and antiretroviral prevention regimes were provided.[64]

The region of Eastern Europe and Central Asia is home to the fastest-growing HIV/AIDS epidemic in the world. An estimated 1.4 million (920,000–2.1 million) people are living with HIV at the end of 2004, which is a ninefold increase in less than ten years.[65] Four features of the epidemic in this region stand out in terms of challenge, opportunity, and hope:

> On the whole, most of the epidemics in this region are still in their early stages—which means that timely, effective interventions can halt and reverse them. Secondly, the vast majority of people living with HIV in this region are young; more than 80% of the reported infections are being found among people below the age of 30 years (by comparison, in Western Europe some 30% of people with HIV fall in that age group). Thirdly, sexual transmission of HIV is increasing in each of the most seriously-affected countries—an indication that the epidemic has gained a foothold in the wider population. Fourthly, ongoing, arduous social and economic transitions serve as the context in which extraordinarily large numbers of young people are injecting drugs. In countries with emerging epidemics demand-reduction programmes that discourage drug use and harm reduction programmes that reduce drug injecting and

prevent HIV transmission through contaminated injecting equipment among young people can prevent larger, more extensive HIV epidemics of the kind now taking hold in Russia and Ukraine.[66]

Clearly there is great need for swift and effective intervention.

Consequences for Development

The presence of HIV/AIDS has catastrophic effects on the infrastructure of nations and peoples. Health care budgets in developing countries cannot begin to address HIV/AIDS because in many cases these countries are not yet able to provide even the basic elements of health care. Fundamental concerns such as potable water, good nutrition, and vaccinations are still major problems in many parts of the world. Many national health care budgets are simply too tight to include funds for the fight against a pandemic such as AIDS.[67] A further obstacle to greater budgetary health care allocation is Third World debt, though at the turn of the millennium there was some success in alleviating the obligations of some of the most heavily indebted poor countries.[68] Repayment plans have had an enormous impact on countries' abilities to set aside more funds for health care.

In the early 1990s, experts anticipated that HIV would undermine overall development in countries most affected by AIDS. Falling life expectancy, large numbers of orphans, economic and business losses due to employee sickness and death, and the destruction of family and community structures were predicted.[69] Tragically, these predictions have come true.[70] HIV/AIDS is the leading cause of death among persons between the ages of 15–59 worldwide.[71] Countries with high prevalence rates are estimated to be losing 1–2% of their economic growth. We see the effects most powerfully in sub-Saharan African countries, where by 2020 the labor forces could be reduced by as much as 35% because of AIDS deaths.[72] The loss of skilled workers undermines a country's capacity to respond to the epidemic. As more educators die of HIV/AIDS, a teacher shortage in several African countries weakens educational systems already challenged by decreasing school attendance and children affected by HIV/AIDS in their families. In addition, growing demands for health care services are overwhelming the already fragile public health infrastructure in many developing nations just as large numbers of health care workers are also succumbing to AIDS. A recent report estimates that in some African countries, AIDS is the cause of death of up to half of all health care workers.[73] A further devastating reality is that the nations struggling most with HIV/AIDS also struggle with malnutrition, food insecurity, and famine.[74] The UNAIDS report declares, "AIDS has become a full-blown development crisis. Its social and economic consequences are felt widely not only in health but also in education, industry, agriculture, transport, human resources and the economy in general. This wildly destabilizing effect is also affecting already fragile and complex geopolitical systems."[75] HIV/AIDS is so devastating to households, communities, and entire societies that responses that would mitigate or remove these effects require local, national, and global efforts and resources.

Prevention, Treatment, and Care

In the years since the epidemic began, most efforts have focused on prevention. Today there is a realization of the integral connection between prevention and care. To be most effective, prevention efforts must be connected with care, treatment, and support. Without this connection, the stigma and discrimination still surrounding HIV/AIDS give persons little reason to learn about or disclose their HIV status.[76] Because HIV epidemics are spreading among a variety of populations even within the same country, prevention efforts must strategically respond to the particular populations. Especially important is reaching out to young people, who are at risk at younger and younger ages.[77]

HIV/AIDS education for prevention continues to be an almost universal high priority, and the area of sex and sexuality is a critical component of such programs. The UNAIDS *Report on the Global HIV/AIDS Epidemic, 2002,* states that "condoms are key to preventing the spread of HIV/AIDS and sexually transmitted infections, together with sexual abstinence, postponement of sexual debut, and mutual fidelity."[78] Even as abstinence is the best way to prevent sexual transmission of the virus, the effectiveness of condoms in prevention has led to tremendous distribution efforts. Research is also continuing on microbicides, in particular non-contraceptive microbicides.[79] Education about HIV prevention for injecting drug users has led to new efforts in this area. Needle exchange programs have been increasing in various parts of the world.[80] The risk of neonatal infection from an infected pregnant woman is significantly reduced for a fetus if proper treatment is available.[81] Today, "prophylactic treatment with antiretrovirals in combination with other interventions has almost entirely eliminated HIV infection in infants in industrialized countries."[82] These efforts must be duplicated in economically poor regions.

Persons are more likely to come forward to be tested for HIV if they know that treatment options are available. A powerful example of this is in Haiti, where voluntary counseling and testing rose by 300% at a clinic where antiretroviral therapy was introduced.[83] This is a prevention strategy because early diagnosis and behavioral changes can limit the spread of the virus to others, prevent reinfection for the affected person, and decrease the spread of other infectious diseases, such as tuberculosis and sexually transmitted infections.[84] Counseling can help people improve their quality of life and support people who are learning to live with their disease.

In June 2001, the United Nations members met in a Special Session of the General Assembly to work out a comprehensive global response to the HIV/AIDS pandemic. The session culminated in a Declaration of Commitment, "a historic landmark" in the fight against HIV/AIDS. This marked the first time that treatment and care, which included access to antiretroviral drugs, were specifically recognized as an essential response by the world's governments.[85] Other important initiatives of the international community have included the Global Fund to Fight AIDS, Tuberculosis and Malaria; the World Health Organization's 3 × 5 Initiative; and the U.S. President's Emergency Plan for AIDS Relief (PEPFAR). In 2004, the Global Coalition on Women and AIDS was initiated in response to the growing number of women infected by HIV/AIDS.

Starting in 1996, when combination antiretrovirals became widely available in high-income countries, the AIDS-related mortality rate plummeted sharply for a few years and has now plateaued in those nations. In Europe and North America, the death rate for HIV/AIDS dropped by 80% in the first four years since the introduction of antiretroviral therapy.[86] Since 2000, there has been greater access to antiretroviral treatment in middle-income and low-income countries. More people have been able to access such treatment because of medicine price reductions for poorer countries. For example, at the beginning of 2000, a year's supply of the combination of antiretroviral drugs for one patient for one year usually cost between $10,000 and $12,000. By the end of 2000, negotiated prices were $500 to $800 for poorer countries, and some generic combinations were as low as $350.[87]

Another significant development is that "generic drug manufacturers in low- and middle-income countries (notably Brazil, India, and Thailand) are producing their own versions of certain antiretrovirals and offering them in their domestic and, in some cases, overseas markets. 'South-to-South' cooperation on drug access is increasing."[88] With Brazil leading the way, an estimated 170,000 people were receiving treatment by the end of 2001.[89]

This good news must, of course, be balanced by the great global needs. Almost 6 million people in developing countries need antiretroviral therapy, and only about 400,000 received it in 2003. This means that nine of every ten people who need treatment are not receiving it. Currently "half of the global treatment needs are located in just seven countries: South Africa (15.8%), India (10.4%), Kenya (6.4%), Zimbabwe (6.2%), Nigeria (6.1%) and Ethiopia (5.0%) and the United Republic of Tanzania (4.1%)."[90] These were among the countries requesting assistance under the 3 × 5 Initiative, which had as its goal the treatment of 3 million people by 2005.

"Living with AIDS" has become an actuality and a powerful rhetorical tool for treatment. A confluence of factors contributed to the reduction of costs for treatment in middle- and low-income countries: "Activist organizations and people living with HIV/AIDS throughout the world have been instrumental in placing treatment-access issues at the top of the agenda . . . dialogue between national governments, international organizations and large pharmaceutical manufacturers; competition from generic drug manufacturers; and legal and diplomatic action at national and international levels" have led to increased access.[91] However, although there are continuing efforts to make treatment prices affordable, the cost remains widely prohibitive to any but those in the United States and other high-income countries.[92]

Global funding has increased to an estimated $6.1 billion in 2004, but the needs are even greater. UNAIDS projects that $12 billion will be needed in 2005 to "effectively respond to HIV/AIDS epidemic in low- and middle-income countries; by 2007 this will rise to $20 billion."[93] Although international donors will provide the most funding, affected country governments have key roles to play. Because almost every region, including parts of sub-Saharan Africa, has countries where the epidemic is still at an early stage or low level, the epidemic can be curbed with effective prevention strategies and interventions. The United States is also a key global partner in the response to HIV/AIDS. In fiscal year (FY) 2005, the "U.S. federal funding commitment for global HIV/AIDS, as part of PEPFAR, is expected to total $2.7 billion, including funding for prevention, care, treatment, and research. This also includes contributions to the Global Fund of $347 million for FY 2005 and a carry-over of $87.8 million from FY 2004."[94] However, much more remains to be done.

FOUNDATIONAL ISSUES BEHIND THE PANDEMIC: GENDER INEQUALITY AND POVERTY[95]

Information about the transmission, demographics, prevention, and treatment of HIV/AIDS is an important starting point for further inquiry. Underscoring this background material are key questions: What are the factors behind the methods of transmission? Who is transmitting HIV to whom? Who is making choices and who is without choices in prevention? In treatment? What conditions promote incidents of transmission? Emerging from these questions are some of the foundational issues that must be addressed if HIV/AIDS and the conditions that make HIV/AIDS more likely are to be eradicated.

African theologian Teresa Okure addressed these issues in a paper delivered to a theological symposium on HIV/AIDS held in Pretoria, South Africa, in 1998.[96] Okure asserts that two viruses more dangerous than HIV enable this virus to spread rapidly among the most vulnerable in society. The first is "a virus which affects people's minds and their cultures . . . It is the virus which makes people look on women as inferior to men—and it affects women as well as men."[97] This virus spurs on the sex industry, in which young girls become HIV-infected and then pass the virus to others, including their own infants. This virus is also "responsible for the shocking fact that in many countries of the developing world the condition which carries the highest risk of HIV infection is that of being a married woman!"[98] According to Okure, one other virus makes possible or even encourages the spread of HIV and is found mainly, though not exclusively, in the developed world. It is "the virus of global injustice which is causing such terrible poverty in many parts of the developing world."[99]

Okure is not the first to name the inferior status of women and poverty/global economic injustice as key issues which must be wrestled with today.

Statistics show that the vast majority of HIV/AIDS cases are in developing countries, where adequate health care resources for the poor, who constitute the greater numbers of people, are generally scarce and sparsely funded. Among others working from this perspective is physician anthropologist Paul Farmer, who writes about women, poverty, and health, and who considers the individual and structural causes of disease and the impact on all involved.[100] Theologian Lisa Sowle Cahill writes about the "survival strategies" people living in poverty are often forced to adopt, which expose them to health risks such as HIV/AIDS. In addition to gender and economic issues, she also discusses the justice lacking in the "interlocking local and global economic systems that disrupt traditional societies, displace economic and educational infrastructures, and cut off access to kinds of prevention and treatment of disease whose efficacy in Europe and North America is well established."[101]

Cahill's remarks parallel those of Richard G. Parker, secretary general of the Brazilian Interdisciplinary AIDS Association, who, in a speech to the 11th International Conference on AIDS in Vancouver in 1996, affirmed that by focusing on social vulnerability it is possible "to more fully comprehend the consequences, with regard to HIV infection and AIDS, of the sexual stigma and discrimination so often faced by gay men or sex workers, of the gender power relations and gender oppression so often faced by women, or of the social and economic marginalization faced by the poor."[102]

In a discussion of why young African women appear to be so prone to HIV infection, several factors common to women in many other countries were mentioned:

> Women and girls are commonly discriminated against in terms of access to education, employment, credit, health care, land and inheritance. With the downward trend of many African economies increasing the ranks of people in poverty, relationships with men (casual or formalized through marriage) can serve as vital opportunities for financial and social security, or for satisfying material aspirations. Generally, older men are more likely to be able to offer such security. But, in areas where HIV/AIDS is widespread, they are also more likely to have become infected with HIV. The combination of dependence and subordination can make it very difficult for girls and women to demand safer sex (even from their husbands) or to end relationships that carry the threat of infection.[103]

Food insecurity fuels the HIV epidemic among women and other marginalized groups: "Bereft of food, people are compelled to adopt survival strategies that might further endanger their lives. Some migrate, often to urban slums, where they are likely to live in marginalized circumstances and lack access to education and health facilities (including HIV prevention and care services). Women and children are being forced, as a last resort, to barter sex for jobs, food, and other essentials. Large numbers of children are leaving school to find work or forage for food. Communities and social networks are breaking down. HIV/AIDS thrives amid such social displacement and disintegration."[104] These are societal conditions desperate for intervention, both immediate and long-term.

The Joint United Nations Programme on HIV/AIDS, under executive director Peter Piot, M.D., has initiated many studies and projects acknowledging and attempting to address some of the local and global sociocultural, economic, and political factors that limit a person's options for reducing their HIV risk.[105] To involve men more fully in prevention efforts, a two-year "Men Make a Difference" World AIDS Campaign was begun in 2000. By focusing on the role of men in the epidemic, this campaign acknowledges that "all over the world women find themselves at special risk of HIV infection because of their lack of power to determine where, when and how sex takes place" and addresses the cultural beliefs and expectations that have led to this situation.[106] The special circumstances that place men at high risk for contracting HIV and the male violence that further fuels the spread of HIV are described, but the balance between "recognizing how men's behaviour contributes to the epidemic and recognizing their potential to make a difference" is emphasized.[107]

Cultural and gender beliefs about fidelity and even violence are a central concern. Many married women and other women in long-term monogamous relationships are not protected from HIV or violence. On April 30, 2004, Dr. Sadik, special envoy of the UN Secretary General for HIV/AIDS in Asia, stated that "the majority of married women who have the infection have had no other partner than their husbands."[108] Statistics reveal that the comments of Okure and Sadik are true for many parts of the globe.

The power differential between men and women takes a toll on women's self-perception. The latest Zambia Demographic Health Survey is a powerful example. For 5,029 women interviewed countrywide, the following statistics emerge: about 80% find it acceptable to be beaten by husbands "as a form of chastisement"; 79% said they should be beaten if they went out without their husband's permission; 61% said a beating was acceptable if they denied sex to their husbands; 45% said a beating was in order if they cooked "bad" food; 88% of women felt their husbands could have sex with them just after giving birth; 67% said they would have sex even though they did not want it.[109] In terms of one form of direct HIV prevention, "only 11% of women believed that they had the right to ask their husbands to use a condom—even if he had proven himself to be unfaithful and was HIV-positive."[110] Clearly, more grass-roots educational work must be done on multiple levels.

Because the AIDS epidemic is increasingly affecting women and girls, the focus of the 2004 World AIDS Campaign, with the slogan "Have you heard me today?" was to raise awareness about and help address the main issues affecting women and girls with regard to HIV and AIDS. What is certain is that many girls and women are vulnerable to HIV because of others' high-risk behavior.[111] Early in the epidemic, the numbers of men infected with HIV far outnumbered the number of women, but today, globally just under half of all people living with HIV are female. The epidemic is affecting women worst in areas where heterosexual sex is a dominant mode of transmission. In a message on World AIDS Day 2004, Dr. Peter Piot named the challenging realities for girls and women and offered some steps needed to halt the epidemic:

> Half of all women live on less than US$2 a day; illiteracy rates among women are nearly 50% higher than among men in many countries; only a small fraction of land is owned by women; and inheritance laws and criminal laws make it easy for men to take advantage of women. Each of these realities makes women more vulnerable to HIV.
>
> We need to give girls everywhere a chance at education, and petition governments around the world to enable women to own and inherit property. Women who are economically self-sufficient and secure are far less vulnerable to HIV. We need to get laws passed everywhere that make domestic abuse illegal, that treat rape as a real crime to be punished harshly.
>
> To reverse these inequities we must focus attention and resources on increasing access to prevention and treatment services for women.[112]

The Millennium Development Goals, which arose from the UN Millennium Summit of September 2000 and declared a commitment to stop and begin to reverse the global spread of HIV by 2015, includes the following: "to halve global poverty; ensure primary-school education for all; promote gender equality and empower women; and reduce children mortality while improving maternal health."[113] The 2001 Declaration of Commitment is a response to unequal socioeconomic development opportunities, economic deprivation, and gender inequality in many parts of the world.[114] And although each nation will have to find ways to respond to these situations within its own context, the global challenge and responsibility are clear. In this age of AIDS, "Many of the world's more marginalized countries also need long-term international solidarity, cooperation and financial support. More equitable investment and trade flows can help ensure that global economic progress also profits the world's poor."[115] A truly global community demands global efforts.

THE ROMAN CATHOLIC CHURCH AND TRADITION

As a universal church, members of the Roman Catholic Church live and worship across the globe. The magnitude of the HIV/AIDS pandemic requires the Roman Catholic community to act on both local and global scales. Indeed, it is the Church's responsibility to act in the face of such a worldwide crisis. And, as it has done in so many ways in other contexts, the Church does offer a hopeful and compassionate response to those persons infected and affected by HIV/AIDS.

Well before the emergence of AIDS, the Church worked across the globe in health care, education, and social services. Through clinics and hospitals, elementary and secondary schools, colleges and professional schools, orphanages, homeless shelters, counseling services, food distribution centers, and much more, the Gospel mandate to love and serve one another is incarnated wherever the need arises. Direct service with and among the people gives the Church a particular competence in speaking to policy issues that directly affect the people of God. The term "people of God" includes all, regardless of religion, gender, race, or ethnicity. Advocacy and direct involvement in efforts on behalf of justice are part of the Church's mission throughout the world. Thus local, regional, and global efforts, especially on behalf of and with those in great need, are part of the Church's ministry, and all people of goodwill are invited to join these efforts. The Church also joins existing common efforts.

In this age of AIDS, the Church has remained with and among the people in areas deeply affected by the human and structural crises that continue to burgeon. The Church's efforts to respond to the AIDS-infected body of Christ include offering access to HIV/AIDS education and treatment and care for persons living with and affected by HIV/AIDS. Organizations such as Caritas International bring together vast resources to deal with the crisis on a local and international scale. Embedded in these actions are not only social service competencies, but also a tradition of faith that treasures the inherent dignity of each person and values the person from the beginning to the end of life.

The theological tradition of Roman Catholicism brings forth its resources in response to the HIV/AIDS pandemic. Catholicism offers a rich tradition, flowing out of the biblical call to love God, neighbor, and self and calling us to lives of fidelity and justice. The Church is also a dynamic institution, bringing its teachings to the world and passionately engaging with the world. In the midst of the AIDS pandemic, the Church has been called to positively offer its theological resources to the people of God. The Church is also being called to probe more deeply into its own tradition as it responds to the signs of the times and the challenges of AIDS.

Three examples of the tradition's dynamic engagement with an AIDS-infected world are found in discussions about (1) prophylactics for HIV prevention, (2) needle exchange programs, and (3) gender inequality.

According to Church teaching, sexual intercourse is to happen only within marriage and is to be open to the unitive and procreative dimensions of sexual expression.[116] In an age of AIDS, sexual abstinence would be the expectation and surest preventative measure for the sexual transmission of HIV/AIDS. The importance of sexual chastity and fidelity within marriage is also clearly stated in church teaching. Thus in global prevention measures, the prevention strategy with the acronym "ABC" finds resonance with church teaching in both A–Abstinence, and B–Be Faithful to one partner. Programs abound in seeking to encourage and support persons in abstinence until marriage, and fidelity within marriage. Yet in the midst of firmly endorsing sexual chastity, what of circumstances in which people, particularly women, are in situations where they do not have free choices for abstinence or are at risk because of a partner's lack of fidelity? The discussion and challenge then is in the discussion of C–Condoms as an HIV/AIDS prevention measure.

The Church teaching on prophylactics in the context of HIV/AIDS prevention has had to consider distinctions between the use of prophylactics to prevent new life and the use of prophylactics to prevent death. For example, some of the debates in the Roman Catholic Church about prophylactic use have centered on concerns that approving such use "could be construed as approving or promoting illicit sexual activity and therefore could compromise Catholic teaching and confuse the faithful; and, second, condoms do not work effectively enough."[117] Such statements have provoked a plethora of responses, from inside and outside the theological community.[118] Although a number of theologians assert that condom use is a necessary prophylactic measure, most also acknowledge that such use is not wholly effective.[119] It should be noted, however, that in July 2001 the National Institute of Allergy and Infectious Diseases of the National Institutes of Health, USA, offered "the largest analysis of published, peer-reviewed studies looking at the question of condom effectiveness" and concluded that although condoms are not perfect, when used correctly, consistently, and under the proper conditions, they do offer significant protection.[120]

While supporting fidelity within marriage and advocating abstinence until marriage, some theologians employ the principle of material cooperation when choices are made for nonmarital sexual activity or sexual activity within marital commitments when one or both spouses are HIV positive.[121] If abstinence is advocated first and foremost, but the persons nonetheless choose to be sexually active, the principle of material cooperation offers a venue for safety, encouraging people to live and supporting life-long growth in a commitment.[122]

The U.S. bishops have spent a great deal of time on questions concerning prophylactic use and have even shifted positions, as can be seen in the two AIDS documents published by the U.S. bishops in the late 1980s: *The Many Faces of AIDS* (1987) and *Called to Compassion and Responsibility* (1989).[123] In *The Many Faces of AIDS*, written by the United States Catholic Conference (USCC) Administrative Board, the board tolerated prophylactic use as one, though insufficient, measure for preventing HIV/AIDS. Debates soon arose among the bishops in light of concerns that condoning condom use would seem to promote uncommitted sexual activity and the use of prophylactics to prevent pregnancy. The second letter, issued in 1989, refrained from any advocacy for prophylactics for HIV prevention. Many theologians have entered this important conversation, and bishops conferences across the world have also studied and spoken on this topic, with varying conclusions.[124]

Needle exchange programs have also been discussed in terms of material cooperation. While not advocating injecting drug use, needle exchange programs provide drug users an HIV-preventative measure while also promoting education, counseling, and assistance for drug abuse treatment. This also helps stop the spread of HIV among users, since needle sharing is not uncommon. Needle exchange programs have encountered some resistance among various members in the Church because some perceive a potential double message of approving illicit drug use.[125] Community debate and resistance, often in areas where needle exchange programs have been run, have also been due in part to concerns about where the drug users would use and potentially discard their used needles.

The Church's rich social tradition advocates justice in all areas of life, and gender inequality is one area of injustice illuminated by the reality of AIDS. The Church speaks eloquently of women's rights in areas such as education, freedom of religion, economic opportunity, and participation in civic life. Increasingly, however, the institutional church is being advised to re-examine its internal practices of justice and equity regarding women if its external calls to gender justice are to be credible. The Catholic community has a crucial role to play in advocating for respect and responsibility among spouses and within all relationships; consequently, its practices are called to greater accountability and transparency. These are but a few of the ongoing discussions in which the theological tradition intersects with HIV/AIDS.

Framework for a Theological Anthropology Needed in a Time of AIDS

To the rich and dynamic Roman Catholic theological tradition, I offer my efforts in the area of moral theology. I ask: What kind of moral theology is needed for an age of AIDS? What kind of moral theology must we engage in, in a world where we encounter HIV/AIDS? I am certainly not the first to ask this question or enter this conversation. For Enda McDonagh, eschatology and the kingdom of God are concerns.[126] McDonagh's question is: What is our image of the kingdom of God in this time of AIDS? Similarly, Kevin Kelly has written on the type of sexual ethics we need in a time of AIDS.[127] To these two efforts, I add my contribution, a constructive proposal for the theological anthropology we need in a time of AIDS.

I begin with theological anthropology because our vision of what it means to be human is crucial and even foundational for HIV/AIDS prevention, care, and treatment efforts. Theological anthropology brings to the fore our Christian tradition and how we see ourselves as humans in light of a relationship with God and relationships to one another and ourselves. The "signs of the times" in our age of AIDS indicate an impoverished vision of the human. The commodification of women and children in so many societies exemplifies this depleted view of life. Cultural conditioning of males that discourages fidelity in relationships also typifies this dearth in anthropology. The dire circumstances of so many living in poverty around the globe illustrate the need to see the human as more than we currently do. How we address this anthropological gap is significant, for it affects self-understanding and individual relationships and choices. The anthropology promoted has significant effects on social, governmental, cultural, and ecclesial institutions, all of which can affect inequalities and structural injustices.

This book is but a beginning and an outline of the very necessary conversation and work needed in the area of moral theology. The crisis of AIDS affords us a powerful opportunity to engage the rich resources of the theological tradition in the service of humanity and exemplifies the challenges that the Church and world face today in responding to the pandemic. The hope is that this book may offer some directions and outlines for moral theology in a world where the body of Christ is HIV+ and the people of God have AIDS.

QUESTIONS FOR REFLECTION AND DISCUSSION

1. Which statistics and demographics did you find most surprising?
2. Find the most recent information for the country in which you live (see UNAIDS at http://www.unaids.org).
3. Look up the most recent available information for the city or state in which you are living (see either http://www.cdc.gov or http://www.state-healthfacts.org).
4. Gather data on a country that interests you and is in a hemisphere opposite yours (north or south) (see UNAIDS at http://www.unaids.org). Share your findings.
5. Read all of the components of the UN Millennium Development Goals (see http://www.un.org/millenniumgoals). Find out the current status of the goals.
6. In what ways has the Roman Catholic Church and tradition been involved in the pandemic of HIV/AIDS? What is encouraging? What further questions do you have?

CHAPTER 2

Toward a Fundamental Theological Anthropology in This Age of AIDS

If we are to respond to the signs of the times today and offer hope, AIDS calls us to look deeply at our fundamental moral theology. Specifically, the situation of AIDS today demands an exploration of our theological anthropology, for how we understand what it means to be human, and what humans need to survive and thrive, will determine how we understand and respond to this pandemic. The AIDS crisis requires a theological anthropology, because we can see from the foundational factors that are contributing to the pandemic that something is gravely wrong with the way we are relating to one another. Something about the human person is not being addressed, is not being held up as being of great worth. Gender inequality and structural injustice cry out for a hopeful response, and theology offers one.[1]

Theological anthropology, a foundational discipline in Christian theology, is concerned with understanding the meaning of human existence.[2] Theological anthropology characteristically deals with "human self-transcendence, the experience of grace, creaturely limitations, and irreducible qualities and capacities of human persons."[3] This brings us into conversation with the human experience of suffering, bodiliness, and hope. Since we are speaking of a theological and even a Christian anthropology, the meaning of human existence must be understood within the context of Christian revelation.[4] Thus, we must bring to our anthropological discussion the insights and resources of the Christian tradition. In particular, natural corollaries to social ethics, moral theology, sexual ethics, ecclesiology, liturgy, and pastoral theology must be considered. Theological anthropology engages the question of who we are in relationship to God, to one another, and to ourselves. Theological anthropology gives us insights into what is integral to our humanity and can help determine our HIV/AIDS prevention and treatment efforts.[5]

A theological anthropology in this time of AIDS calls for an understanding of the human person as a *relational, embodied agent* in a context of *suffering* and *historical realism.*

Suffering is the point of departure for theological anthropology. Suffering must be the starting point for any theology in this age, for it is a reality that must be named and addressed in all ways, including theologically. Following a discussion of the reality of and resistance to suffering, I move to an exploration of historical realism, our embeddedness in history and society.

Again, these theological anthropological elements are not exhaustive. They suggest what needs to be further developed if we are to practice fundamental ethics today and effectively respond to the AIDS crisis. The elements underscore the person as relational in both particular and general contexts, with a dynamic nature that invites growth toward the divine, the other, and the community. They are also useful for considering other contemporary moral and social issues. Theological anthropology is a lens from which to engage the signs of the times.

In naming the elements of a theological anthropology that is most helpful in a response to HIV/AIDS and its relationship to gender inequality, poverty, and structural inequality, several sources are engaged, especially those of feminist, liberation, moral, and political theologies. One source, however, merits special mention.

While not necessarily offering foundational insights provided by each element of the proposed theological anthropology, Johann Baptist Metz emerges as a consistent and grounding conversation partner in several ways. Metz's theology addresses the situation of suffering in the world in terms of both a stance and an invitation to action. His powerful experiences as a youth in Hitler's army, the Holocaust, and the paucity of writing on it by (European and German) theologians, including his mentor, Karl Rahner, led to Metz's conviction that one cannot do theology with one's back to the Holocaust.[6]

Nor, I contend, can theology of any sort, and especially fundamental ethics, be done with our back to the modern plague of AIDS. As a Christian theologian, Metz brings a theological perspective to his understanding of the human person and engages questions that flow from experiences such as genocide, pandemics, and plagues.

Metz engages those who feel that nothing is to be done in cases like AIDS, who feel that "It's hopeless, so let's despair or deny." In response to suffering, he grounds his activity in the deep roots of the Christian tradition, which are connected to a community of believers. He sees hope, a "solidaristic hope," in the struggle even if solutions are not immediate. His is a faith and theology and Christianity for the long haul. Metz offers a *stance* from which to live and act that operates on a multiplicity of levels. This stance impels one to be with the suffering other even as one pushes for changes in structures. In the midst of suffering, Metz also acknowledges a relationship to God that addresses affliction and includes hope. His is a resurrection-oriented theology which, while not denying the anguish of passion and death, affirms a hope within which one acts—the Reign of God as here and not yet here.[7]

Metz resists the privatization of religion, stating that our Christian tradition calls, invites, challenges, and compels us to respond to the other in need.

Immersion in one's faith has a necessary corollary to one's *active* involvement in the world sociopolitically. Metz asserts that "any theology which tries to reflect on Christian traditions in the context of world problems and to bring about the process of transference between the kingdom of God and society is a 'political theology.'"[8] Thus, "religious" or "theological" activity will have an eschatological character. In all this, Metz offers the beginning of an ethics of discipleship that I will further develop in later chapters.[9]

SUFFERING: REALITY AND RESISTANCE

The starting point for any discussion of AIDS must be the experience and reality of suffering. If theological anthropology explores the meaning of human existence, it must encounter the reality, the voices, and the faces of human suffering. One need only read the newspaper, watch the news, or listen to stories of the marginalized and oppressed of society to begin to see wholesale suffering. It includes bodily, psychological, emotional, and spiritual suffering.[10] Such suffering exists in the midst of and stems from experiences of poverty, violence, repression, and oppression.[11]

A certain consensus has been reached among political, liberation, and feminist theologians around the globe; that is, one must begin with experience, the experience of poverty or radical oppression and repression in various parts of the world, and especially underdeveloped countries. From a variety of disciplines, these theologians give voice to and attempt to respond to suffering in similar yet nuanced ways.[12] Here we will specifically attend to those realities that are direct or contributing factors in HIV/AIDS and are included in the previous chapter.

We begin with two dimensions of suffering: the reality of suffering rooted in experience, and resistance as a response to suffering.

Reality Rooted in Experience

The starting point for Edward Schillebeeckx's theology and ethics is the experience of disorder. It is disorder, on personal and social levels in our world, which has damaged and continues to threaten human beings. So that the privileged few may profit, the vast majority of humans suffer. The masses suffer "exploitation and oppression or rejection, not only from individual human beings, but above all from sociopolitical, economic and bureaucratic systems, anonymous forces which are nonetheless real."[13]

Theologian Patricia McAuliffe introduces her work, *Fundamental Ethics: A Liberationist Approach*, with a similar claim: "Our experience of the world is not one of harmony, order, a God-given plan. Rather it is overwhelmingly one of disharmony, disorder, suffering, oppression. People are being destroyed due to their class, sex, sexual orientation, color, religion, language, because they are 'too' old or because they are 'handicapped' . . . other species and the environment are being destroyed because they are seen as mere means to some people's ends."[14] McAuliffe puts flesh on the victims of various "-isms" in society. Certainly the statistics and demographics of our first chapter speak to this reality.

African American theologian M. Shawn Copeland names some of the painful emotional limits and edges that unabated suffering brings. She states that "suffering always means pain, disruption, separation, and incompleteness. It can render us powerless and mute, push us to the borders of hopelessness and despair."[15] This is the suffering to which theology and theological anthropology must respond in order to restore self-determination, voice, and hope to the individual and to the community.

Liberation theologians writing from Latin American experiences particularly hone in on historical suffering and oppression. Ignatio Ellacuría, whose own suffering and fate mirrored those of the people whose lives he wrote about, describes the reality of the people of God as "the existence of a vast portion of humankind, which is literally and actually crucified by natural oppressions and especially by historical and personal oppressions."[16] Both Ellacuría and Sobrino turn to the crucified Christ in order to convey the reality around them. For both, the cross serves as a poignant and powerful image, a Christian symbol that is a historical reality and a present-day reality for too many. Sobrino uses the cross as an image of the suffering of the poor and describes the primary reality of the world as widespread suffering.[17] He writes that material deprivation and emotional impoverishment become mutually reinforcing, strangling experiences.

Sobrino challenges the First World and the First World Church: "To actually do away with this suffering is the way of salvation for both Third and First Worlds . . . [S]tated simply, the task of theology today, either in the First or Third World, cannot be carried out if the massive, cruel, and mounting suffering that pervades our world is ignored. If a theology closes its eyes to suffering because such suffering is not occurring massively in 'its' world, that theology would disassociate itself from the real historical humanity in which we all live and which, theologically, is God's own creation."[18] Sobrino declares that from the point of view of liberation theology, "theology has to be done within a suffering world, because such a world is the most real world," and in Latin America and for most people today, "poverty is a massive reality."[19]

This is a sizable challenge for First World churches and communities, for even in our domestic and local communities it is much easier and more comfortable not to face the situation of AIDS. Yet, by definition, being "Catholic" connects us with the universal Church, a Church that daily encounters the neighbor and family member with AIDS.

Metz has a strong preferential option for those who suffer, and he locates authority among those who suffer. He believes that "there is one authority recognized by all great cultures and religions: the authority of those who suffer. Respecting the suffering of strangers is a precondition for every culture; articulating others' suffering is the presupposition of all claims to truth. Even those made by theology."[20] Metz locates God's authority in those who suffer, "stressing a respect for and obedience to the authority of those who suffer. For me this authority is the only one in which the authority of the sovereign God is manifested in the world for all men and women."[21] Metz reminds us that we cannot be a Church and do theology without meeting the faces of HIV/AIDS and responding with our personal, social, and global resources.

Resistance as Response to Suffering

Our discussion of resistance as a response to suffering considers three areas. The message of the cross as a central Christian symbol must be understood as a stance of fidelity and love and as a stance against suffering. In a brief exploration of Jesus' life and ministry, we will recognize a complete *no* to human suffering. Finally, we examine two powerful forms of resistance that have been used in times of intense struggle: lamentation and sass.

For many theologians, resistance—open-eyed resistance—is the appropriate response to suffering. Schillebeeckx names such resistance to suffering "negative contrast experiences," experiences of negativity on both a personal and a societal level which cause human beings to be critical of human suffering and to act against that suffering, in anticipation of a better future.[22]

Metz also advocates a resistance to suffering and describes this resistance theologically, personally, and sociopolitically. Using a phrase from Peter Rottlander,[23] he writes that the sole content of Christianity's universal responsibility is that "there is no suffering in the world that does not concern us."[24] J. Matthew Ashley, commenting on Metz, suggests that the "limit-situation" that Metz brings out in distinguishing authentic ways of being human "is the presence of meaningless suffering and death *of the other*, the histories of suffering which characterize this history in which we exist and become subjects (as being-in-history) at least as much as the histories of growth and attainment of freedom."[25] The way we must meet this limit-situation is to acknowledge, resist, and remove suffering.

The Cross

Any discussion of suffering must address the cross as a central symbol of Christianity. Since crucifixion is the means by which Jesus of Nazareth died a painful death, the cross certainly speaks of suffering. But what does the cross say about suffering?

A response to suffering in the world must include at least an initial discussion of the cross for our time and place.[26] Mary Catherine Hilkert reminds us that "Christians never had only one understanding of the cross; it is far too profound to be explained by any one theological perspective."[27] Writing on the topic of preaching on the cross, she continues: "Nevertheless, contemporary preachers are called to preach on the mystery of the cross in a specific time and culture. What aspects of that mystery are forgotten in our day?

How might traditional doctrines be heard in the context of massive global suffering and by the suffering members of the Christian churches?"[28]

As Christians who claim that Jesus Christ offers a model of what it means to be fully human, surely we must have some insight into suffering and resistance to suffering if we consider the life, death, and resurrection of Jesus. Acknowledging that there is a need for a critical appropriation of the mystery of the cross, Hilkert states: "the last word about the cross may be that it is indeed a mystery of divine love, fidelity, and solidarity, but the first word that must be spoken is of its scandal, injustice, and absurdity."[29]

The cross is first and foremost a scandal. The cross was "a weapon of execution, a form of capital punishment," and "considered from the point of view of history, Jesus was an innocent man who was unjustly executed."[30] The crucifixion is not to be considered God's will in any sense, since it was not God but human evil and injustice that brought Jesus to the cross. To understand the cross, Jesus' death must be seen in the context of his life and resurrection. It is "not suffering and death that is redemptive. Even the death of Jesus is salvific only in the context of his life and resurrection."[31] Paul's letter to the Corinthians reminds us that the cross without the resurrection would be worthless: "If Christ was not raised, your faith is worthless" (1 Cor 15:17).[32] Schillebeeckx suggests that "in one sense we are saved in spite of the cross, rather than because of it."[33] Not suffering, but "a love that was fierce enough to triumph over the forces of death and evil and a compassion that was broad enough to encompass all of creation" is what saved us.[34] We will fill out this picture in later chapters, but it is important to remember that "in the end Jesus faced the cross as the final consequence of fidelity to his preaching mission with a radical hope in the compassionate God he knew as Abba. He filled an experience that was in itself meaningless and absurd with meaning, love, and a sense of solidarity with all the innocent who suffer. What Christians celebrate is not the cross, nor the sufferings of Jesus, but the power of a love that is faithful even unto death."[35]

It is crucial that we not glorify or romanticize suffering or the cross. Boff both cautions and asserts that "[t]he cross always crucifies . . . To preach death and the cross in a genuinely Christian manner is to invite our fellow Christians to embrace this powerful, revolutionary love, which is an identification with sufferers such that we actually join them in their struggle with the mechanisms that produce crosses. What we must *not* do is preach death and the cross for their own sake."[36] Ellacuría and Sobrino aptly remind us that in a world of "not just wounded individuals but crucified peoples," enfleshing mercy, which is a task of Christianity, means doing everything we can to bring the crucified people and peoples down from the cross.[37] This is Jesus' *no* to suffering.

Thus in resisting we may suffer; we may suffer because of a connection, a relationship in some way to the other who is suffering. We endure suffering not for its own sake, but because the goal or end is to alleviate in some way, if not remove, the suffering of the other. Our resistance and resulting suffering are essentially an incarnational interruption into the reality of the suffering of another. Confronting the suffering of persons with or vulnerable to HIV/AIDS may put at risk our First World comforts and economies. Yet, both love and justice call us to place ourselves where gender inequality and poverty lie, to allow ourselves to be transformed by these realities and to transform those factors that allow these injustices to exist.

Jesus' Life and Ministry

Even as the cross is the central element of our Christian tradition, we must remember that the cross is not without a history. Jesus' life and ministry help us understand the prelude to the cross. Hilkert offers a number of reasons why Jesus died on the cross:

> Jesus was executed as a political criminal and a religious blasphemer as the consequence of his "dangerous preaching" of the Reign of God. His healing ministry and his inclusive table companionship threatened traditional boundaries that distinguished insiders from outsiders in both religious and political realms. Jesus shocked religious authorities as he announced the forgiveness of sins, a proclamation that was the prerogative of God alone. He touched lepers and spoke with Samaritans. He formed bonds of friendship with women and tax collectors who collaborated with the oppressive Roman Empire and invited both into the circle of his disciples. A faithful Jew, he radically reinterpreted Jewish tradition and laws of Sabbath observance and ritual purity. His liberating lifestyle, his shocking parables and beatitudes, and the unconditional compassion of God that he embodied in his person and style of relating were all profound challenges to religious and political structures of the day.[38]

We cannot forget that even today in some settings persons with HIV/AIDS still bear a stigma akin to that of leprosy; that many are outsiders because of gender, ethnicity, or economics; and that many are judged by religious communities to be sinful failures. How welcome, then, is Jesus' example of embodied love. In the midst of suffering and debasement, being met by a community of believers who follow this incarnated love would be a sign of great hope.

Jesus spoke and acted from a love that threatened the status quo because that love so fully celebrated the gifts and potential of all and excluded no one from the fullness of life. Jesus' message was to set free all those who were imprisoned and oppressed; the full force of this mission was clear as he read the words of Isaiah, declaring that the spirit of the Lord was upon him to bring glad tidings to the poor, to heal the broken-hearted, to return sight to the blind and to announce favor from the Lord.[39] These words are as dangerous as they are freeing, for they upset the given order. Significant relational changes are implied, and a clear sense of God's care and love for God's people is transmitted. Jesus' message was utterly freeing and relational.

Jesus, whose entire life declared "God's 'no' to our suffering in history,"[40] offered immeasurable possibilities for all people, a dangerous proposition in a hierarchical society with significant differences in social status. He saw no need to imprison people in a poverty that denied love, acceptance, forgiveness for human frailty, new beginnings, or food, shelter, and clothing. Jesus' life is a *no* to the concepts of a First and a Third World, to privilege, to domination of one person or group by another, to a rejection of the other because of gender, sexual orientation, religion, class, status, or place of birth. Jesus' message was for the one and the many. This is the full humanization of each, which is essential for the humanization—the full humanity—of all.[41] When Metz and Rottlander proclaim that the suffering of any one is the suffering of all, their message has an obvious corollary in the life of Christ. We must acknowledge that in our First and Third Worlds, where economic, social, and gender inequalities exist, no one is truly liberated and all are essentially imprisoned. The call is to recognize this essential imprisonment and to respond to the suffering of any and all. For when the body of Christ has AIDS, we are all somehow carrying HIV.

Lamentation and Sass

Resistance as a response to suffering can take any number of forms, for the human spirit's capacity for creativity is endless. We will briefly consider lamentation and sass. Both responses of resistance are relevant to persons directly oppressed and those seeking to end the suffering of others. Both lament and sass are also part of the larger process of restoring right relationships among individuals, in society, and in religious institutions.

As a form of resistance, we lament because we hope. Metz reminds us of the power and importance of lamentation. He retrieves the strands of the lamenting tradition, which includes the prophets, psalms, and the books of Lamentations and Job.[42] These strands "call God to account, grumble against God, but also expect more of God, expect more of history, and thus empower and require those who hear and enact them to *act* more out of those apocalyptic hopes and expectations."[43] Since the master narrative for Christians is the dangerous story of Jesus' suffering, death, and resurrection, it is at the cross that one also hears the poignant lament, "My God, my God, why have you abandoned me?"[44] We need to stand silently at this place, yet in our own stories "the embrace of pain through the process of lament is possible, however, only because one has hope that the future can indeed be different. Grief that is not despair is rooted in a memory of a past that has been lost or changed, but also in a future that can be imagined if not remembered. The hope of the paschal imagination is that death, injustice, and loss do not have the final word; the future lies in the hands of the living God."[45] Thus we lament the 3.1 million men, women, and children who died of

AIDS in 2004. We lament at the cross of the 39.4 million persons living with HIV/AIDS. We lament the 4.9 million newly infected with HIV during 2004. We lament because we hope; and we imagine a future that can be radically different from this reality. We lament because we hope; and we actively seek to have our hope realized despite and in the midst of a daunting pandemic.

Sass is another form of resistance.[46] Through an exploration of the narratives of enslaved and fugitive Black women, M. Shawn Copeland examines the language of sass as a form of resistance to suffering.[47] Three points are crucial. First, through the language of sass women named their experience and their reality. Women who had no power in their society used language to speak their reality and truth, to defend themselves against physical, sexual, and psychological assault, and to claim their moral authority. Copeland writes that women used sass "to guard, regain, and secure self-esteem; to obtain and hold psychological distance; to speak truth; to challenge 'the atmosphere of moral ambiguity that surrounds them,' and, sometimes, to protect against sexual assault."[48] Notably, in women's slave narratives the women describe themselves "not as passive subjects, but as active agents who make whatever decisions are possible to take charge of their lives and to resist brutality."[49]

Where did this resistance come from, when so often the Christianity preached in the South offered one standard of moral living for the white planter class and another for slaves? Copeland notes that Christianity was a fundamental resource for Black women in resistance, but that women drank selectively from its well.[50] A second point, then, is that the women resisted a Christianity which in any way tried to assert that suffering and bondage were God's design for them. The language of sass resisted stories of the cross as a symbol of submission and instead saw the results of the cross as a triumph over evil. Spirituals about the cross of Jesus were empowering and encouraging, for "the enslaved Africans sang because they saw on the rugged wooden planks One who had endured what was their daily portion. The cross was treasured because it enthroned the One who went all the way with them and for them."[51] Scripture, particularly the book of Exodus and the Gospels, held out hope of a future far different from their present situation, and this hope came forth in sass. Third, sass allowed the women to name their reality, appropriate their faith tradition properly, live in hope, and pass on to their children memories of and hopes for liberation. Sass could certainly result in further physical violence and even death for the women, yet speaking out their truth had a power of resistance that the women did not otherwise have.[52]

Suffering must be the starting point for any theology and for any responsible and effective response to the situation of AIDS in our world today. The suffering described above is deeply rooted in the reality of the world and in an experience of a God who is not absent from but in the midst of this encounter.

EMBEDDEDNESS IN HISTORY AND SOCIETY—HISTORICAL REALISM

Any personal or social response to a humanitarian crisis must flow from an understanding of our embeddedness in history and society. To this we now turn as our second necessary anthropological element.

Metz claims that an authentic understanding of what it means to be human is one that is firmly embedded in history and society.[53] One and all are part of and formed by both history and society. We are both historical and social human beings, and we understand ourselves through our history and within our society.

As North Americans and as members of the "First World," we have access to the entire globe in ways unparalleled in previous generations. Such accessibility is our distinct advantage and challenge. Like others before us, we can reflect on human experience through a variety of empirical, analytical, and theoretical sciences. However, our range of reflection includes even greater access to cultures and societies beyond our own. With worldwide availability of information, a sense of our place in history can also be more global.[54] When we see ourselves connected historically and on a scale larger than our national borders, we understand that a U.S. response to AIDS must be more far-reaching than a prevention and treatment plan for our own country.

To be human means to be connected somehow to a history and to a society. We are born in particular times and places and learn about who we are in our specific historical settings. Although our embeddedness is particular, we can choose to be either more parochial or more global in our awareness and engagement of our historical, social, and cultural circumstances. As an individual, the responsibility I take for this is contingent upon my vision and the vision of my community.

What does expanding one's vision of history and society require of us? Three immediate responses present themselves to us. The first requirement is a stance of openness as we become aware of the historical and social realities that make people and societies vulnerable to HIV/AIDS. The second requirement is to name our locus for structural transformation. Here we are seeing with open eyes, allowing this reality to permeate and to critically and creatively engage our faith. The third requirement is active engagement in the processes of transformation. This level of response flows from individual transformation and engages the larger community and institutions and structures. It is primarily a communal way of life. Openness, a willingness to see, and active engagement are the requirements and the risks of being fully human. Let us explore these further.

Listening and Seeing: Historical and Societal Levels of Poverty and Oppression

Metz reminds us that there is a constructive level to an understanding of ourselves in history and society. This is the productive, dynamic, evolving nature of our being human. However, Metz argues that the "meanings which we construe and construct, in which we come to recognize ourselves, are fragmented. Our being-in-the-world as subjects is equally threatened and fragmentary. Any interpretation of the meaning of human being cannot be gained at the cost of covering over this fragmented, endangered character of historical experience."[55] Metz reminds us of the underside of history, where being a subject and understanding one's meaning in history and society are challenging. Such is the dark side of our history and society, for those who lost rather than gained, where life diminished for people rather than offered opportunities for flourishing. Metz's concern for human historicity and temporality as constitutive dimensions of human existence led him to notice and respond to those areas the writers of history (i.e., the winners) often choose not to remember, or mention only briefly. For Metz, in post–World War II Germany, the issue was the Holocaust. For us today the issues include AIDS and dire poverty on local and global scales.

Seeing our history and society through the eyes of the poor is part of the first requirement of listening. The admittance of the poor into the consciousness of all has been a key concern from the earliest days of liberation theology. In recent years, African liberation theology has offered insights that push conversations about poverty and the poor from individual poverty to national, regional, and continental poverty. This in turn challenges wealthier nations and transnational corporations to an examination of practices and policies that contribute to poverty across borders.

African theologian Engelbert Mveng writes of poverty in the Third World, notably in Africa, as an anthropological and structural phenomenon.[56] Noting that material poverty, "more often than not, produces misery—the state of absolute indigence in which a human being, deprived of everything, lives in conditions at times inferior to those of an animal," he adds that material poverty is often inseparable from spiritual, moral, cultural, and sociological poverty.[57] This anthropological poverty is an "indigence of being."[58] Poverty, in turn, not only affects individual and social groups, but also greatly affects the state, "that symbol of power, independence, and sovereignty. It makes a political vacuum of the state, which in turn wafts above a dark, apocalyptic void: the economic vacuum . . . A subjugated state can be neither a state of rights nor a paradise of liberties. Deprived of both political and economic sovereignty, such a state is helpless to ensure the development of its citizens."[59]

In looking at various causes of impoverishment, Mveng moves to a consideration of structural sin, both within African nations and within the global community. He considers both the agents of impoverishment ("incarnations of violence and oppression") and their victims ("the mass of the poor, the weak, the oppressed, and the disinherited, those without voice, without right, and without power") and calls this impoverishment "political."[60] This political impoverishment corrupts—at their very roots—the interpersonal relations of human beings so that they become relations between powers. It culminates in the anthropological and political poverty that we call structural poverty.[61]

Naming the Locus for Transformative Engagement in History and Society

In this section we explore two guides the Christian faith tradition offers for reflecting on the world around us: the Good News and the common good.

The Good News

As a response to "world domination by those who possess force, wealth, and power," Mveng proposes "evangelical poverty," which lies in the imitation of Christ as the "great mobilization for the establishment of the Reign of the Beatitudes throughout our world."[62] How will this happen, this access to evangelical poverty for Third World persons? Mveng's answer is clear and challenging to persons, communities, and institutions:

> *The only answer is that they must first themselves be free.* That is why, in the face of the structures of sin and the factories of impoverishment and misery, the evangelization of the Third World—that is, the proclamation to that world of the good news—demands first and foremost the destruction of the structures of sin and their spawn: the factories of power, misery, and the vicious circle of impoverishment. The political and economic order of the world today is an arrogant challenge thrown in the face of the church. The church can no longer worthily accomplish its mission without a radical reassessment of the political and economic order and the structures of sin that guide the world. It is not enough merely to bring down the Jericho walls that are the structures of sin. The most important thing is to replace them with counter-structures, whose mission is not only to neutralize the effects of the structures of sin but, especially, to mobilize the Christians of the Third World to follow Christ the Liberator and themselves become liberators of their sisters and brothers.[63]

African theologians are trying to articulate a way of being human which acknowledges the need for both the poor and rich to see together a new vision of humanity. Their writing is situated in their particular social, cultural, and historical situations; yet the message resounds for the entire global community.[64]

African liberation theology implicates and challenges the Church. Jean-Marc Ela from Cameroon begins his essay "Christianity and Liberation in Africa" with the declaration that the "concrete, historical irruption of the poor in our midst poses questions for our faith today" and explains how this challenges African Christianity.[65] However, the poor in our midst are a challenge to Christianity everywhere. Instead of being treated as basic rights, "access to drinking water, a balanced diet, health and hygiene, education, or self-determination are, more often than not, luxuries for a self-serving club" in many African nations.[66] Clearly, the Church's justice efforts to ensure basic human rights for all are integral to prevention and treatment strategies, not only for HIV/AIDS, but for many other forms of human suffering.

Ela also places Africa on the cross when he writes bluntly: *"Africa today is crucified.* An African theology that rereads the Bible in terms of this fundamental locus will have to be a 'theology of the cross.'"[67] Placing the Scriptures in the midst of the grim situation in Africa, Ela asserts: "We must take account of our situation that is the result of the joint enterprise of the multinationals, the cozy smugness of the ruling classes, and an all-pervasive corruption. When we view this situation in the light of the central mystery of our faith, that wellspring from which we draw the strength to forge ahead, the first thing we discover is the prophetic character of the poor and the other marginalized groups who, by their very existence within our societies, manifest the nature of sin in its historical structure."[68] Christianity is directly challenged to look and see and not simply continue on its way, "passing the victim lying in the ditch."[69] Ela is undoubtedly aware of internal factors contributing to the dispossession of the masses.[70] However, he challenges the Church, first and foremost, to take up the causes of oppression and injustice.[71]

This is a challenge for the entire church, both in Africa and beyond. Citing the example of Jesus, Ela reminds Christians that Jesus' preaching was not limited to an internal conversion. Liberating the poor and oppressed was also Jesus' concern (Luke 4:16–21). Ela wants the Church to do more than incorporate African rhythms and words into the liturgy; he challenges the Church to learn the conflicts of African history and to live Christianity in terms of the present historical and social dynamics of Africa.[72] Thus African reality "imposes on the church a kind of *pedagogy of the discovery of situations of sin and oppression*—situations that rear their heads in contradiction with the project of the salvation and liberation in Jesus Christ."[73] For the resurrection to be more than a simple event of the past, for the incarnation to continue in a world of such suffering and conflict, the people of God must be open and willing to listen deeply to the experiences of those who live in these conditions. As people the world over are reading Scripture in light of their actual experiences, the challenges of poverty, oppression, and AIDS provide the historical context in which the church must listen, live, and act.

The Common Good

Lisa Sowle Cahill brings the historical and social realities of the global AIDS pandemic and its structural agents of transmission[74] into conversation with the resources of Catholic social thought.[75] She focuses on the common good as an avenue for dynamic engagement with local and global signs of the times. Cahill acknowledges that the individual behaviors upon which HIV infection depends, particularly sexual contact and IV drug use, must be addressed. However, she believes more attention must be focused on the

social conditions that influence these behaviors, as well as on the social circumstances which can promote changes in behavior patterns.[76] While
acknowledging that 90% of people infected with HIV live in underdeveloped and developing countries, her analysis includes the gaps in care in the
United States and other affluent countries.[77]

The common good is inherently connected to another key tenet of the
Catholic tradition—justice—which is "the association of person in community according to relationships and structures that serve the common good
of all."[78] This principle asserts that "every member of society has a right of
participation in the common good, claiming rights and fulfilling responsibilities; the ultimate purpose of the common good is to enhance the well-being
of every single member of society, as well as of society as a whole. The common good includes both the material and the social aspects of human flourishing."[79] Actualizing our principles of Catholic social teaching is yet another
resource for the transformation of structures which make persons vulnerable to HIV/AIDS.

Active Engagement in Processes of Transformation

In this section I offer examples of women working toward the transformation of society in South America and Latin America. It is important to
remember in this discussion that within any society and culture there
are a variety of histories and groups struggling to speak from the margins.
The experience of women in most societies is that of the margins, and this
marginality can exist simultaneously in Third World and First World societies. In their concrete histories and societies women are struggling for
liberation.

Writing from one of the poorest sections of her country, Brazilian theologian Ivone Gebara notes the movement in which women are challenging
the cultures that consider women inferior to men and oppression against
women to be acceptable. This "irruption of history into the lives of
women—and especially the theological expression of their faith— . . . is,
the irruption of historical consciousness into the lives of millions and millions of women, leading them to the liberation struggle by means of an
active participation in different fronts from which they had previously been
absent."[80] Gebara offers a powerful image and description of this irruption:

> It is as though a strong wind had begun to blow, opening eyes and loos-
> ening tongues, shifting stances, enabling arms to reach out to new em-
> braces and hands to take up other tools, impelling feet to take other
> steps, raising the voice so its song and its lament might be heard.
> Woman begins to take her place as *agent of history*. The fact is that with
> her activity and new stance toward what happens in life, a new aware-
> ness is clearly coming into being. Entering into history in fact means
> becoming aware of history, entering into a broader meaning, in which

women are also creators or increasingly want to be forgers of history.[81] [emphasis mine]

Participation in labor unions, neighborhood movements, mothers' groups, and pastoral leadership manifests a change in the consciousness and in the role women play today.

This historical awareness, coupled with an engagement of Scripture and one's faith in the circumstances they encounter, has moved women toward a greater sense of their ability to respond to and to engage a history and society that are changing and changeable. Luz Beatriz Arellano of Nicaragua writes that basic ecclesial communities brought to light a new image of the spirituality of women, transformed from a passive spirituality to committed women reading the Scripture in terms of their life experiences and in terms of a new responsibility, a new ability to respond, within history.[82] She writes, "Galatians 3.28 is becoming something real, since women are finding that they are protagonists in history, history-making subjects liberating themselves and liberating their people."[83]

These examples are hopeful stories of the journey, of the Reign of God that is here and not yet. These are stories of women who "discovered that no one was going to liberate us from outside. We discovered that the Lord was really present within us, and this impelled us to change our own situation."[84] These are women and men who, in sharing their stories of passion, pain, and joy, united to create and transform situations of oppression. Not all stories are those of success, however, at least not in the present. Too many stories continue to unfold of the poor being unable to gain access to proper drinking water, without which they cannot even consider taking medicine for malaria or HIV. Too many newspaper accounts of violence toward women and children continue to be found. Too many stories continue to be told of torture of those naming structural injustices.

Yet we must continue to tell the stories of the community gathering for a common good. Arellano writes of the integration that began within her community between the God of life, Jesus as *compañero* (colleague, fellow revolutionary), the Church as community, and the building of the Kingdom of God.[85] Such an integration led to a vision of church that not only questioned itself internally, but that also took responsibility for all on the margins. This led to questions about how to announce the Good News of Jesus with deeds and not simply with words. The group began to "take on small tasks aimed at transforming society."[86]

QUESTIONS FOR REFLECTION AND DISCUSSION

1. Why is it that "The starting point for any discussion of AIDS must be the experience and reality of suffering"?
2. When have you known suffering? What was its root cause? What stories of suffering have others shared with you? What was its root cause?

3. What is the connection between suffering as reality and resistance and the cross? What does this have to do with HIV/AIDS?
4. What stories of lamentation and sass are you familiar with? Do you know of any stories of lamentation or sass that have emerged from nations or cultures or other large groups? Are there any being voiced aloud today?
5. Recall the first time you became aware of poverty or oppression.
6. Recall the first time you saw a situation "through the eyes of the poor." Who taught you? What images were present?
7. What are some examples of an "irruption in history" that led to freedom from suffering? What might an "irruption in history" look like for God's people with HIV/AIDS?

CHAPTER 3

Embodied Relational Agent

A theological anthropology in this age of AIDS includes an understanding of the human person as an embodied relational agent.[1] I will first consider the agent, then the agent as relational and finally as embodied. The three concepts are integrally related, and the discussion of one term will invariably include the other terms. However, for the purpose of more clearly and carefully describing our vision of the human person, I will consider them separately. The terms are precisely the missing and misunderstood elements of the human person in today's AIDS struggle—for purposes of prevention, for commitments in relationships, for globally and locally addressing the pandemic's foundations. Our sexual and social ethic has not yet fully grasped the multifaceted dimension of the person in this way. My effort is to probe these elements a bit further. This section is essential for considering gender inequality and the dignity of all persons as well as evaluating the sexual ethics we live by today.[2]

AGENT

Essential to any vision of the person is that one is an agent. The *person as agent is a dynamic subject with participatory and self-determining capacities for living out one's loves and desires.*[3] To see exactly what this might mean, I will separate the interlocking terms of this definition.[4] The agent as *subject* is in opposition to person as object. "Object" removes the person from the heart of decision-making, and "subject" defines the self to be a central starting point for discernment and decisions.[5] The agent is a "subject" who acknowledges the inherent and integral good of each person and the dignity with which each person is to be regarded and treated. In addition to being the starting point for decisions, the agent must have self-determining capabilities for discernment and decision-making. Without this, the agent has no reason to continue.

Acknowledging a *capacity for self-determination* gives meaning to choices and commitments. Self-determination necessarily flows out of freedom. Commitments can be freely chosen and with respect for oneself as well as for the other(s). This freedom for self-determination is not disembodied, without social context, personal ties, or history.[6] It is instead a freedom *for* relationship and *in* relationship. Self-determination affirms responsibility in relationships and considers the complexities of decisions. The moral agent is to "act according to his or her conscience, in freedom, and with knowledge," and the "other" is also to be respected as an agent "capable of acting with the freedom of an informed conscience."[7] Self-determination requires that one is an active, engaged, and free *participant* in discussions and decisions.[8] Self-determination requires freedom, including a free and informed conscience. But what is the purpose of the agent's freedom and self-determination?

Quite simply, agency exists for the sake of *love*. It is about the love of self, God, and the other, in a continually spiraling movement. Love ultimately extends to all of creation. Only the agent as self-determining subject can answer the question: "Who will I love and how?" Loving oneself, knowing oneself as loved by God and an other(s), as well as loving another and God and caring for oneself, are all part of agency. There is an activity and a receptivity in this description. The agent freely chooses loves out of her *desires*. The agent in freedom is situated. Margaret Farley offers a helpful description of the interrelationship between our freedom, desires, and loves:

> Freedom is not opposed to desire (as Kant thought it was), but desire is not in the first instance free. Shaped as we are in the fabric of our lives, our desires rise not from our free choice, but out of what we already are—including our needs and loves, fears and hopes, deprivations and fulfillments. These desires, rising unbidden, nonetheless present themselves to our freedom. Our desires mediate for us the options of freedom. For whenever we are confronted with alternative possible actions, these actions become viable choices only if we desire them in some way.
>
> But desires have not only a history; they arise not only out of the past that has generated some deeper affective response; they rise out of our loves. Loves, too, have a history, and they rise unbidden by our choice. But, like the desires that express them, loves present themselves to our freedom. Every action that we choose is for the sake of some love, whether for ourselves or for another, whether for persons or for things. When we choose our actions, we ratify, identify with some of our loves (deferring, or refusing to ratify, other loves that are thereby not expressed in action). And the same is true for the desires that come from our loves; we affirm some and refuse to affirm others, letting the ones we affirm issue in action or commitment to action.[9]

The agent is also a *dynamic* subject, capable of growth and a deepening of one's loves and commitments and actions. Just as cultures, societies, and institutions are capable of change and therefore growth,[10] so too is the person. Farley offers a useful connection between freedom and growth. "Freedom, then, is possible not in spite of our loves and desires, but because of them—because they express who we are and present what can be chosen, because they do not always compel us to remain as we are. Becoming truly one with our loves, and in that process shaping them—sustaining or changing, strengthening or weakening, integrating or fragmenting—that is the possibility and the task of our freedom. Freedom then rises out of relationality and serves it. Freedom is for the sake of relationship—with ourselves and with all that can be known and loved."[11]

The dynamic nature of the person allows for an incredible possibility for good in relationships and situations that the agent as subject can incarnate. While realizing that every person is capable of failing to love, the dynamism I propose here essentially focuses on the person's capacity and activity of love.[12] Seeing the person as dynamic acknowledges the present reality of the person and appeals to the best that one is and can be. The dynamic character of the agent offers time and room for growth.[13]

Agency thus speaks deeply to all layers of relationship and calls us to respond to our loves. We now move to the second part of this chapter, a closer examination of the person as relational.

RELATIONALITY

Modern U.S. society has created a division between the individual and the community that essentially limits a vision of the person who can respond to the situation of AIDS on both a personal and communal level. We now explore a few theological images from Latino, African, and feminist voices which contribute to an understanding of the person as relational and which affirm the individual and the community.

Roberto S. Goizueta writes, "where there is no strong, constitutive sense of community, then the relationship between the particular (individual) and the universal (family, church, community, tradition, institution) will appear intrinsically dichotomous," and modern liberal individualism will opt for the individual against the community.[14] For U.S. Hispanics, "there is no such thing as an isolated individual who is not intrinsically defined by his or her relationship to others . . . [T]he entire cosmos . . . is an intrinsically relational reality where . . . each member is necessarily related to every other member. The person, therefore, is always *intrinsically* relational."[15] This sense of community extends to ancestors as well as progeny for Goizueta[16]; the same is true for Metz's understanding of community and for various African communities. Goizueta further writes that the working anthropology for U.S. Hispanics is that of a Jesus who is a physical, historical reality identified and defined by concrete, personal relationships—with his mother, his followers, his beloved, and us.[17]

Goizueta is also one of many who cite the Trinity as an indication of the relational character of God and human persons.[18] Mercy Oduyoye sees the unity in diversity of the Trinity as a helpful model for relationships among individuals and the community. She writes that "we find the Persons in constant and perfect mutual relationship and we are reminded of the need for properly adjusted relationships in our human families, institutions, and nations."[19] The distinctiveness of each person and yet the unity or community created among people is the model she suggests for further application in church and society. Margaret Farley grounds "agape"[20] as mutuality in Trinitarian language and asserts that a human love typified by mutuality and equality best exemplifies the quality of relationships within the Trinity: "the First Person and the Second Person are infinitely active and infinitely receptive, infinitely giving and infinitely receiving, holding in infinite mutuality and reciprocity a totally shared life."[21] Relationality here includes the possibility for trust, intimacy, honesty, and commitment.

LIFE OF THE BODY

We now consider the person as embodied. A fuller and theological understanding of the body is crucial for any understanding of AIDS—for ways in which the Church can respond to caring for the body before it has AIDS as well as when it has AIDS. We relate to ourselves, one another, and God through our bodies. Our bodiliness is essential, not optional or mere garnishment. The body is the way through which we know and express ourselves as physical, emotional, psychosexual persons. Yet, it is precisely these areas that are compromised for women and other vulnerable populations in many parts of the world. There is power and freedom and vulnerability in knowing ourselves as embodied; and perhaps more than in any other area of theological anthropology covered so far, more is at stake here in this age of AIDS. It is to our global peril if we disregard the importance of understanding our bodily selves as sacred.

We turn now to a discussion of embodiment through four categories: history of the body, sources of sexual inequality in the Christian church, emotions and voice, and sexual expressions of the body.

History of the Body

In an excellent historical survey of Christian attitudes toward the human body, James Keenan reflects on Scripture and tradition to highlight the appreciation of the body, which is rooted in the Incarnation. Countering popular belief that the Church has always held a negative attitude toward the human body, Keenan cites numerous sources to illustrate how the Christian tradition "has always regarded the body as constitutive of human identity, and some strands of that tradition have vigorously combated various expressions of dualism."[22] The body as "object" emerged in the Enlightenment and can be seen as such in medical writings and procedures from that period.[23] S. Kay Toombs writes: "Medicine has, for the most part, adopted a 'Cartesian' paradigm of embodiment . . . The physical machine-like body is assumed to be extrinsic to the essential self."[24]

However, the human body described in Scriptures and throughout early, medieval, and Renaissance history is always a person, a subject.[25] Scholars such as Steinberg and Bynum make it clear that "the gender-specific depictions of Jesus do not accentuate his body's gender but rather demonstrate the full integration of the body of Christ."[26] Keenan summarizes this well, stating that "just as Christians labored to understand the unity of Christ as fully human and fully divine, no less have they attempted to understand themselves as fully one in body and soul and in the body of Christ. That is, the challenge of Christian revelation in Christ incarnate is to overcome dualism, fragmentation, and division both in our anthropology and in our ecclesiology."[27]

Sources of Sexual Inequality in the Christian Church

In the midst of a reemerging appreciation for the body as a whole, issues of gender and gender inequality must be addressed. In her article "Sources of Sexual Inequality in the History of Christian Thought," Margaret Farley asserts that "Christian theological traditions have too easily found ways to establish 'equality before God' for both women and men and a simultaneous 'inequality before one another' which accepts a hierarchical relationship precisely on the basis of sexual identity."[28] While in early Christianity the shared grace of baptism offered a moment of freedom and equality, two fundamental roots of sexism in theology are the identification of women with evil and the identification of the fullness of the *imago Dei* with male persons.[29] Farley lists several tasks for the Church that are relevant if gender inequality is to be uprooted. These include understanding the body and sexuality outside the realm of defilement and sin, understanding human weakness and human strength as part of the human condition of *all* persons, and reconstructing the doctrine of *imago Dei*.[30] Both the history and the present understanding of the body offer us insights into the center of the tradition and the growing edges of the tradition.

Emotions and Voice

Contemporary psychology and theology have reminded us that our emotions are embodied and even stored in our bodies if we do not immediately attend to them.[31] One of the ways intimacy is communicated is through emotions and voice. We are integrally connected to our feelings. Our feelings are communicated in any manner of nonverbal expressions. Our joy and fondness for another can be expressed through a hug, a kiss, or a smile. We can express sorrow or anger through tears or by throwing rocks in the ocean. Emotions are powerfully conveyed through voice, inflection, and narrative. There is great power in one's voice, for through voice the body speaks, and with it comes information from all parts of the body—mind, emotion, spirit.[32]

The power of voice can be illustrated through an example of violent silenc-ing of voice. In *The Body in Pain*, Elaine Scarry writes that torturers work to make the victim cry out not only in pain but in submission through self-blame. Torturers exact power by tearing the voice from the body of their victims: "The goal of the torturer is to make the one, the body, emphatically and crushingly present by destroying it, and to make the other, the voice, absent by destroying it."[33] The body is left voiceless. Scarry "highlights that silencing and other forms of exclusion are physically and personally destructive acts, but that the body as subject finds its expression in the verbalized narrative."[34]

This is precisely why the voices of women and all those on the margins of AIDS—children, minorities, gay men, non–First World peoples, the poor—must be attended to, why they must be heard.[35] Our stories, our shar-ing of intimate and personal parts of our lives, are part of what it means to be embodied human persons. We are our voices, and honoring and pro-moting the verbal expression of persons is part of our nature.

Sexual Bodies/Sexual Expressions of the Body[36]

Finally, essential to understanding the human person before God is an understanding of ourselves as sexual, with bodies capable of incredible inti-macy. Every person is a sexual being, and the way that we express our sexu-ality depends on a variety of factors, including the nature of our relationships and commitments. While there are many ways of defining "sexuality," a helpful description for our use is the following: "Sexuality is love energy. It refers to the spiritual, emotional, physical, psychological, social and cultural aspects of relating to one another as embodied male and female persons. Sex-uality, a still-evolving term, has to do with all the ways we try to reach one another at the level of the heart. It involves our efforts to communicate, our acts of tenderness, and even our struggle to find each other again after an argument. It is the constantly burning fire within us that compels us to turn toward one another. In this sense, we are being sexual—expressing our rela-tional energy as women and men—all the time."[37] This fire within us is in search of intimacy, with ourselves, with one another, and with God. As sex-ual beings what we seek most, and throughout our lives, is intimacy.

In his book on sexual ethics and AIDS, Kevin Kelly reminds us that "our sexuality enables us to share a very special kind of intimacy with another per-son—not just physical intimacy, but a more fully integrated personal inti-macy. That profound intimacy can be celebrated, communicated, shared and enjoyed in a very unique way through the highly symbolic physical act of sex-ual intercourse."[38] Sexual intimacy in a variety of forms can be moments of embodied love and healing in a relationship. We love, argue, hurt, and heal as bodily persons, so it makes sense that all of these can be done through sex-ual expressions.

The premise in considering the sexual expressions of our bodies is that inti-macy lies at the heart of the relational dimensions of being human. As such, sexual physical intimacy, including genital intercourse,[39] is one way of mutu-ally sharing love energy and is meant to be pleasurable.[40] Genitality[41] is a very important and vibrant way of expressing intimacy, but it cannot be the only or even the main expression of intimacy, even in a committed relationship. There are many layers of intimate expression that are part of maturing and growing relationships.[42] The invitation and challenge in the physical sexual expressions of intimacy in relationships is to ask how this expression is deep-ening one's love for oneself, the other, and God. Thus, sexual intercourse should always be at the service of intimacy, and not vice versa.[43] In all of this, the body as positive, as the conduit of the Incarnation, must be clearly communicated.

In marriage, the unitive dimensions of sexual intimacy include openness to the procreative dimensions. At the end of Vatican II, *Gaudium et Spes* (Pastoral Constitution on the Church in the Modern World) offered several important points on the meaning of marriage and family life. Two in par-ticular are important to mention here. First, intimacy in marriage is described in terms such as "community of love" and "intimate partner-ship of life and love" (#48). Second, while not asserting a "hierarchy of ends or goals," marriage and married love are also "ordained for the pro-creation and education of children" (#48). Parents are to see themselves as "cooperators with the love of God the Creator, and are, so to speak, the interpreters of that love" (#50). The call is that through the Christian fam-ily, "which springs from marriage as a reflection of the loving covenant uniting Christ with the Church" and "by the mutual love of the spouses, by their generous fruitfulness, their solidarity and faithfulness, and by the lov-ing way in which all members of the family assist one another," all will see "Christ's living presence in the world" (#48).

There are many challenges to advocating an understanding of the sexual body as has been described above.[44] In many media contexts, sexual inter-course has become not an expression of deep intimacy but a physical form of relating that does not presume other forms of intimacy between persons. Physical elements are highlighted at the expense of relational and emotional contexts. The Catholic Church has consistently voiced its teaching that sex-ual intimacy requires the context of a committed relationship, but for many, this message is lost in negative messages about sexual expression that the Church has at various times also advocated. Teaching about intimacy has at times been lost in the teaching about genital expression. Kelly and others remind us that a revised sexual ethics is needed that "makes faithful sexual loving *attractive* to people and is based on values accessible to the thinking of ordinary men and women. If such a sexual ethic could be articulated in sufficiently positive language, it might help in limiting sexual intercourse to faithful sexual relationships. This would not be due to any fear of AIDS, nor because of being constrained by any external pressure from Church teach-ing, but because of the attraction of such a life-style if it is seen to be the way to achieve the greatest happiness as sexual persons."[45]

Violent sexual contexts are a significant factor in the spread of HIV/AIDS among many women. Examples of violent contexts for women include but are not limited to stranger rape, coerced sex from committed partners, unsafe conditions for sex workers,[46] lack of power to demand that a sexual partner use a prophylactic, and unsafe sexual intercourse with someone, even in marriage, who suspects that he has the virus whether or not the person is tested. When sexual intercourse occurs and even one person objectifies the other, at worst the *imago Dei* is not at work, and at worst the people of God are on the cross again. All of this has everything to do with "our dignity as human persons made in the image of a relational God."[47] Essential here is a positive view of the body and the sexual person that allows one to move toward the other in intimacy and at the same time to grow and to deepen one's relationships.

QUESTIONS FOR REFLECTION AND DISCUSSION

1. What area of embodiment have you found to be most at risk in society today? What would a respect for the body require of you? What would it require of your peers?
2. Relational existence is a key element of being human. What avenues of relation are strong in your generation? What elements are missing?
3. Consider the various elements of agent and agency. What might you add to that description?
4. When have you known relationality and agency to conflict? What helps move the conflict to a resolution that is positive for both parties?
5. Who models a healthy embodied relational agent for you today?

CHAPTER 4

Virtues for a Time of AIDS

How do we live out the theological anthropology of Chapters 2 and 3 in this age of AIDS? The type of embodied relational agent just described needs to develop or cultivate particular qualities, and the virtues name those qualities. Now we will see how the virtues bring our theological anthropology to life.

Virtues are dispositions and habits, which flow out of who we are and who we want to become, and they offer a vision of how to get there. The task of virtue is "the acquisition and development of practices that perfect the agent into becoming a moral person while acting morally well. Through these practices or virtues, one's character and one's actions are enhanced."[1] Lee H. Yearley writes, "a virtue is a disposition to act, desire, and feel that involves the exercise of judgment and leads to a recognizable human excellence, an instance of human flourishing."[2] The virtues are fully embodied, involving the physical, spiritual, emotional, mental, and social capacities.

Virtues are teleological; that is, there is a goal or end toward which they strive. In Aristotle's time, happiness would have been a goal. In Christianity, the ultimate end is union with God, and we live out this desire on a daily basis through our love of God, neighbor, and self. Throughout our lives we strive toward this telos, and as long as we live our task is not complete. Virtues, like our human nature, are also dynamic; therefore, as we continue to learn, grow, and mature, so our level of understanding and depth of living the virtues evolve.

The virtues tell us what is constitutive of the horizon of our expectations, of that place in which human flourishing is realized. The virtues do not offer detailed directions on how to become a certain kind of person, but they do offer a roadmap. In the situation of AIDS today, an examination of some particular virtues offers us a general route, a broad highway from which to respond to AIDS. Five particular virtues I will highlight in this chapter are hope, fidelity, self-care, justice, and prudence.[3] These virtues are discussed in enough detail to provide a description that fits our universal humanity and yet are sufficiently general that they can be modified and applied to every culture.

43

A field of ethics that has taken anthropology most seriously is the ethics of virtue. As Keenan explains, "the virtues are traditional heuristic guides that collectively aim for the right realization of human identity . . . The historical dynamism of the virtues applies correspondingly to the anthropological vision of human identity, which guides us in our pursuit of the virtues. That vision is also, in its nature, historically dynamic. As we grasp better who each human person can become, to that extent we need to reformulate the virtues."[4] Liberation theologians Antonio Moser and Bernardino Leers also point to the historical dynamic of the virtues: "Virtues, like the people who perform them, are not independent of time and space, but take shape and are practiced in specific historical situations."[5] Just as the theological anthropology developed names the identity of the person as that of an embodied relational agent, so too for virtue ethics, "the primary identity of being human is not an individual with powers needing perfection, but rather a relational rational being whose modes of relationality need to be realized rightly."[6] These descriptions of the relational person in turn offer further opportunities for cross-cultural discussions.[7] The virtues invite integration of our personal and communal lives.

While Aristotle's *Nicomachean Ethics* and Thomas Aquinas's discussion of the virtues in the *Summa Theologiae* are certainly seminal texts, much work has been done on the ethics of virtue in the past two decades.[8] Alasdair MacIntyre, Stanley Hauerwas, William C. Spohn, William Joseph Woodill, Joseph J. Kotva, Jr., Antonio Moser, and Bernardino Leers, for example, have all written on virtue ethics from a Christian perspective.[9] Theologians writing on specific virtues include, among others, Margaret Farley on fidelity, Diana Fritz Cates on compassion, Marie Vianney Bilgrien on solidarity, and Christine Pohl on hospitality.[10] Each of these contributions has developed or enriched various virtues and placed them more fully within the moral life.[11]

The work of James F. Keenan, SJ, whose writing on the virtues also considers a relational anthropology, offers a helpful starting point for examining virtues relevant to the situation of HIV/AIDS.

Keenan sought to examine a constellation of virtues that could offer insight into human identity. He settled upon the cardinal virtues after reviewing bibliographical literature that suggested there were many people interested in fidelity, justice, and self-care.[12] Keenan observed at least an implicit consensus about the significant role of these virtues. Along with the virtue of prudence, these three need one another to flesh each other out as they interact. None of these virtues stands alone; rather, each informs, frames, and helps develop and deepen the other as the person grows into virtuous living.[13]

In his article "Proposing Cardinal Virtues," Keenan asserts that all persons are relational in three ways, and that each of these ways demands a cardinal virtue. The term "cardinal" "suggests that all other virtues 'hinge' on these four and, therefore, as such they sculpt the outline of our anthropological vision."[14] We are relational in a specific way, and that requires the virtue of fidelity. We are uniquely relational and thus require the virtue

of self-care. As persons we are relational in general, and the virtue of justice must flow from this. Finally, prudence as a fourth cardinal virtue determines what constitutes the faithful, self-caring, and just way to live.[15]

I will examine each of the cardinal virtues as described by Keenan. However, before doing so, a few further questions about virtues and HIV/AIDS
must be addressed: Can we even consider an anthropological thickening and
an anthropological vision in this time of AIDS? Can we even attempt this,
given the overwhelming number of persons living with HIV/AIDS? Can we
attempt such a vision, given the impoverished and unjust living conditions in
so much of the world today? If we can consider an anthropological vision,
on what basis can we consider articulating an ethics of virtue for a world
with AIDS? The answer to the first set of questions is yes, and we can articulate the ethics of virtue in this age of AIDS because of the essential virtue of
hope. It is hope, then, that we must turn to first.

HOPE

Hope is the virtue that gives us a particular sustained moral vision. In addition, it is the transcendent virtue that animates and informs the virtues which
follow. William F. Lynch's work on hope and the imagination connects imagination quite directly with hope. In linking these qualities, Lynch writes that
the importance of imagination "is not so much that it has vision as it is able to
wait . . . to wait for a moment of vision which is not yet there."[16] Hope not
only gives us the vision, it sanctions and sustains the vision. Christian hope
tells us what type of vision we have. Hope is also a prime Christian resource
of the imagination.[17] Hope points to the telos of Christianity and offers a horizon for our expectations in both tangible and nontangible ways. Hope is the
vision that allows us to reshape our reality in a particular way. Hope imagines
what could be and animates the virtues to bring to life what is imagined.

In addition to a horizon for our expectations, five other points underlie
the virtue of Christian hope: (1) hope is communal; (2) hope includes the
dead as well as the living; (3) hope is connected to help; (4) hope is connected to the paschal imagination; and (5) hope has a fundamentally eschatological dimension.

The communal nature of hope is such that it not only imagines, but *imagines with*; it is inherently collaborative and promotes mutuality.[18] Hope is
an act of the community, whether the community is large or small, global or
local. The community may consist of the nations that follow through with
UNAIDS financial commitments. The community may be pharmaceutical
companies that commit to providing medicine at prices affordable for poor
nations. The community may be a family whose members support one
another in the day-to-day challenges of caring for a relative living with AIDS.
What do these groups hope for? Perhaps they hope for a vaccine or a cure for
AIDS; for treatment for HIV/AIDS; or for the intimacy of a relationship as
they struggle with AIDS.

Since almost 40 million persons around the globe are living with HIV/AIDS today and 20 million others have already died from AIDS, it is especially important that hope include the living and the dead. Metz writes of solidaristic hope, a hope that includes those who have gone before us.[19] As we act out of a horizon of expectation that the dead are part of our energy and drive in seeking a cure for the disease, hope remembers all and leaves no one behind.

Hope is also connected to help. While hope is within us, hope is also the sense within us that there is help outside of us.[20] Lynch writes: "There are times when we are especially aware that our own *purely inward resources* are not enough, that they have to be added to from the outside. But this need of help is a permanent, abiding, continuing fact for each human being; therefore we can repeat that in severe difficulties we only become more especially aware of it."[21]

Hope is integrally connected to our paschal imagination. The life, death, and resurrection of Jesus are a message of hope that does not evade or deny the suffering and dying that occur in life. Yet the crucial and incarnated hope is that the end of the story is not death, but new life, which may take a variety of forms. Imaginative hope does not evade reality, but sees it and transforms it.

Finally, hope is centered on the eschatological nature of our lives as Christians. Our life includes doing all we can to promote the Reign of God in the world. At the same time, our faith tells us that ours is a "here-and-not-yet" reality and that the Kingdom will not be completed in our lifetime. This is not a reason for inactivity, but it once again places our activity in a wider context. Christian hope here is time-attentive and -responsible, but not time-bound. This allows us to work toward the Reign of God and yet rely on God in the midst of it all.[22] Hope ultimately reaches out to all that is good, all that is God.[23]

A scriptural passage intimately connected with hope is the post-Resurrection story in Luke 24:36–40. When Jesus appeared to the disciples, his wounds, the marks of his crucifixion, were apparent.[24] New life, a transformation, had happened, yet not in the way anticipated. Jesus was not expected by the disciples to appear in the room where they were gathered, and especially not with his wounds. Yet the wounds were one of the ways that the disciples were able to recognize Jesus.[25] New life had emerged. For Christians, the paschal mystery is the quintessential paradigm of hope. Hope is the basis from which we take on a fuller way of being human in the midst of a pandemic.

With an understanding of hope as the transcendent virtue that animates and informs the four virtues of fidelity, self-care, justice, and prudence, we will now examine each of these in turn, as they unfold in a similar way. We will begin with a brief general discussion of each virtue, followed by markers for the virtues, which are then applied to HIV/AIDS.

FIDELITY

Fidelity is a virtue of relationship, and, more to the point, of specific relationships. It is the virtue that "nurtures and sustains the bonds of those special relationships that we enjoy whether by blood, marriage, love, or sacra-ment. Fidelity requires that we treat with special care those who are closer to us."[26] By its very nature, fidelity is partial and particular.[27]

The ties that bind us by fidelity are very specific. Such relationships are marked by a deep, abiding respect for the inherent dignity of each person. Fidelity marks the relationship of parents and children. This relationship evolves as children grow and mature into adulthood and continues to evolve as parents age. There are different markers for each of these times in the life of a family, and the call and virtue of fidelity require us to meet differ-ent responsibilities in different situations.

The fidelity that marks a friendship is dependent on the level of the rela-tionship. There is a level of equality and mutuality in friendship that is dif-ferent from that between a parent and child. The fidelity between two per-sons in a committed relationship has yet another level of depth and breadth of mutuality to it, but it, too, is marked by an equality of relationship. In this section I focus on the fidelity that marks the bonds of friendship, particularly relationships of marriage or permanent commitment. HIV/AIDS prevalence would be reduced if interactions within these relationships were marked by fidelity. To this end I examine the virtue of fidelity and offer some markers for such relationships.

As noted by Farley, fidelity is rooted in love.[28] Interpersonal fidelity is about active receptivity, and in love and commitment this means that the "freely chosen commitment of love testifies to the reception of the beloved in the life of the one loving, and by commitment the one who loves yields to the beloved a new claim on his or her love . . . One will be claimed, called, at the disposal of another. But the call of the other is always to the freedom of the one who has made the commitment. Freedom gives to another a claim on itself, but if it can respond to the claim only as freedom, then its new being-bound is not a foreclosure on freedom but a new call to continuing self-transcendence."[29] While this freedom and commitment will often enough call one to sacrifice for the relationship and for the other, this "yielding" is a positive act, for it does not compromise the value of the person "yielding." Instead, it is part of the interplay of persons growing in freedom and com-mitment to one another.

Farley further writes: "to commit oneself to another, to give one's word, is to place oneself in the other in a new way, to yield to the other a claim over one's future free choices."[30] This commitment is at the same time both *binding* and *freeing*. Fidelity also requires a *mutual commitment* to growth. Each must commit to the relationship and to one's own growth as well as to the other's good and growth. This is why fidelity as permanent commitment requires both a great deal of maturity at the onset and a pledge to a lifetime of growth.

Fidelity affirms that persons can achieve selfhood in relation to an other.[31] Here we see again how our theological anthropology, especially including its elements of relationality and agency, is further brought to life through the virtues. We become more faithful, as shown by our lives and actions toward one another in relationship. This fidelity manifests itself in greater intimacy with the other. The commitment to the other in fidelity is a mutual growth experience, even as there will be mistakes on the journey. Over time and with attentiveness to the disposition and practice of fidelity, relationships grow and deepen and become more faithful.

Three significant markers or expressions of fidelity include mutual honest communication, embodied expressions, and consistency.

Fidelity demands honest mutual communication. We must be willing to share what matters most to us. We must also be willing to listen and to hear what matters most to our loved one. Such relationships are marked by deep listening and honest sharing, both of which are the places of our vulnerability and represent our relationship's growing edges. This does not negate disagreements or hurts; yet fidelity is grounded by a willingness to continue coming together and to deepen the level of mutual trust. Fidelity calls us out of our comfort zones to our growth zones. Our heart's workings, desires, and struggles must be communicated in words and emotions. Fidelity is present and attentive even when the other does not speak, in the long moments of silence with one another. In our frenetically busy lives, fidelity is a commitment of our time, in which we intimately share the details of our lives, our narratives, with one another. In our relationships we, like Mary, keep these stories in our hearts and encourage and love another in freedom to grow.

Communication requires that we stay at the table long enough not only to listen to, to hear, and to speak with one another, but also to work through the nuances of decisions that result from mutual sharing. This requires compromise at times. For example, one partner's new job offer might be a graced opportunity to use more of her gifts and to work in a more collegial environment. For the other partner, however, this invitation might mean a loss of net income, a new city in which to adjust, and the need to find a new job as well as new schools for the children. Fidelity requires that the ways in which situations affect each person are discussed. This may also require the compromise of one for the other, which, as long as it does not cause violence to either, is part of the practice of fidelity.

Honest communication in light of AIDS requires that we share our histories with one another. A husband's spouse has the right to know whether his journey has included activity which may not only present a risk to her, but which may present a risk to him and to their mutual well-being. Sexual activity that puts either partner at any risk for sexually transmitted diseases must be discussed. The same is true for injecting drug use or any other risky behavior. Both are sources of HIV transmission that must be addressed in a committed relationship or one moving toward a commitment. As painful as it is, if I engage in risky behavior while in a relationship, fidelity requires communicating this for the safety of the one who may now become infected. Communication is the means by which we seek reconciliation for our mistakes if we are truly repentant. And fidelity requires such honest and vulnerable communication.

Fidelity in committed relationships is also marked by embodied expressions of commitment.[32] To respect the other and to share deeply and intimately is to honor one's own body and the other's body in all ways of relating. Faithfulness in a relationship requires that partners communicate on a variety of levels. Our bodies are the vessels of our love, our anger, our strength, our vulnerability, our struggle, and our peace. The ways we touch one another communicate love or anger, power or mutuality, violence or wholeness/holiness. We must be attentive to all that we communicate, for our bodily expressions tell of our understanding of our relationships.[33]

We must be attentive to the telos from which we begin our sexual relationships, even as we realize that not every single act of sex will deepen a relationship. A sexual understanding of our bodies reminds us that we have sex in many contexts, including love, joy, sorrow, stress, and healing. Our cognitive and affective lives are affected by our intimate expressions with one another, just as our voiced communications are. Fidelity reminds us that bodily expressions are sacred narratives that must be honored as such.[34]

 A challenge in our age is that sex can represent a recourse to power and domination rather than mutuality. When "sex itself is enough," it may be used to circumvent the real and greater need for deep sharing. Sex without a relationship may temporarily cover loneliness and longing, or it may painfully remind us of it. In all this, an awareness of one's own body and of the other's body is a key indicator of the level of a relationship. At various times the union will be more powerful for one than the other, but fidelity demands that there is on the continuum an awareness of the other and his or her needs. Sex and fidelity do not converge when sex regularly satisfies only one person.

A third marker of fidelity is consistency. Fidelity is about the long haul.[35] When we freely, intentionally, and with all that we at any given moment can know about ourselves and the other, make a promise to fidelity, it is a moment of great trust and great risk. Consistency has to do with our presence to one another in terms of time and attentiveness. Consistency is about seeing the other as the main partner through which community with others grows. Consistency is also a faithful response in the midst of a society constantly seeking new stimulation and quick answers. In the midst of frenzied activity, fidelity calls us to attentiveness on a regular basis.

In this age of AIDS, fidelity is a consistent response to the suffering of the other. Here, mercy, the willingness to enter into the chaos of the other's life, is framed by fidelity so that in the relationship each knows the other will not be abandoned in times of need. Consistency here means finding ways to express fidelity safely. The need for intimacy and for intimate touch requires creative ways of loving.[36] Fidelity also asks the partner and caregiver to be honest about limits and to seek and accept help from others.

The consistency and steadfastness of fidelity do not exclude others from joining the community of care.

SELF-CARE

Self-care addresses the unique relationship each of us as a moral agent has with ourself. Keenan reminds us that the virtue of self-care is about our "unique responsibility to care for ourselves, affectively, mentally, physically, and spiritually."[37] In light of the pandemic's focus on women and those on the margins of society, care for the self is essential. Some critics of self-care equate this virtue with selfishness or self-centeredness. These critics claim that self-care excuses people from social justice activism or from any self-sacrifice in the name of justice. This is not the understanding of self-care proposed here. Feminists such as Margaret Farley and Barbara Hilkert Andolsen, among others, seek alternatives to both the strict autonomy model represented in critics' claims and the inappropriate self-sacrifice often encouraged of women.[38] The model of an embodied relational agent discussed in Chapter 2 offers such a balance. Self-care is the virtue that is held in balance with both fidelity and justice. And self-care is crucial for persons vulnerable to HIV.

The virtue of self-care is attentive to the person as *imago Dei*. Created in the image of God, the person is to be treated with great respect and dignity. Both common good and human rights language centers on the innate dignity of the human person and her right to pursue affective, mental, physical, and spiritual well-being and growth.[39] Edward Vacek reminds us of the importance of and interrelationship between love of God, love of self, and love of neighbor.[40] From a consideration of God's love for each of us individually, Vacek reminds us that since we are "most constantly present to ourselves, whose needs we are usually most able to fill, and whose moral self we alone are able to form, we are therefore our own nearest 'neighbor' . . . our love for ourselves is irreplaceable and indispensable. We have talents and a personal identity that we alone can develop. We have a relational self that we alone can enact."[41] Thus, in very integral ways we are responsible for our own lives.[42]

What does self-care look like in a time of AIDS? Three specific markers of self-care in terms of HIV/AIDS are commitment to growth, relationality, and self-acceptance.

Commitment to growth requires a level of self-awareness. I need to know how I am relating to myself, to others, to my God, and to the larger community around me. In reflecting upon this I better understand my gifts and limitations. I may know, for example, that I have a variety of relationships and that certain relationships include expressions of intimacy. I may also be aware that I am not yet prepared to make a permanent commitment to another, even though at some point in the future I would do so.

A commitment to growth sees growth in the long haul and yet responds to the immediacy of a situation. Theologian Roger Burggraeve advocates a growth ethic that is to guide people to a "meaningful sexual life" by providing an "ethical optimum" as a "goal to strive for."[43] Self-care as a commitment to growth is an invitation to positive and meaningful experiences of relationality permeated by the value of the entire relationship, and not simply by the sexual end of the relationship. Such an ethics of growth and commitment to growth must employ language rich in positive images of continual growth and encouragement to growth. Self-care is thus promoted in images and acts. Growth into fidelity and permanent commitment invites abstinence in a very positive manner. Fidelity to the other I am coming to know more deeply is essential.

Yet what does one do in an age of AIDS in which young people in particular are making choices that nonetheless put them at risk for HIV/AIDS? Burggraeve writes of an ethics of growth as an ethics of mercy.[44] According to Burggraeve, once the "ethical optimum" has been offered as well as possible, a commitment to growth must include safety measures for the other and for myself. While the ethical optimum must still be encouraged, the "ethical minimum" provides for the basic dignity of the persons involved and for the prevention of HIV infection through both "just sexuality" and the "principle of equality."[45] While this is intended to prevent the transmission of HIV, Burggraeve clearly states that this is neither an adequate sexual ethics nor a starting point for Christian ethics.[46]

Burggraeve argues that prophylactics and, in a similar vein, needle exchange programs, offer opportunities for at least minimum self-care and harm reduction. While the person is taken as she is in her situation, there is always an invitation to more growth and maturity.

Relationship is a second marker of self-care. Self-care requires that one be in relationship, not only with oneself, but also with others. We care for ourselves when we develop significant, positive, supportive relationships. Healthy, positive relationships, community supports, and a relationship with our God are crucial elements of self-care. In this age of AIDS, community supports are ways of both connecting with and grounding ourselves. Responding to God's invitation to relationship is a way of caring for myself, since realizing the spirit of God within me is essential for seeing myself as *imago Dei*. And to find *imago Dei* within myself is to recognize myself as good and holy.

Persons on the margins of society and at risk for HIV infection may not easily find supportive relationships or community supports. Self-care requires supportive relationships because there are times when we all need to lean heavily and depend on others. The poor Indonesian woman, the gay Hispanic male, the sex worker desperate to support her family, the spouse whose husband refuses to reveal his HIV-positive status when asked about the lesions on his body—all of these people must find supportive relationships that will affirm their goodness and encourage them to take actions to protect themselves. On whom will these people on the margins lean for comfort, support, endurance, or healing? On which communities can they depend? All of us

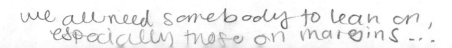
we all need somebody to lean on, especially those on margins...

must find people and spaces in which to safely lean on them. Self-care is about how we take care of ourselves, and this includes allowing others to care for us. The support of a Source and community is essential if we need to leave unhealthy commitments and relationships that cause violence in our lives. Supportive relationships assist us in growth and healing.

A third essential marker of self-care at this time is self-acceptance. Self-care, which includes awareness, desire for growth, and life-giving relationships, engages our gifts and our limitations. Self-care encourages each person to reach a level of peace with his or her essential self. People outside the margins are rarely encouraged to do this, yet it is necessary. When a person becomes HIV-positive, society still stigmatizes the person with the infection. Just as a person with cancer cannot be defined by his disease, a person with HIV cannot be defined solely by the infection. In some countries an HIV diagnosis means the person is removed from the family support system. In some relationships "HIV-positive" means one will never again be held. This denigration may be internalized as self-loathing, and self-care may be replaced by risky and unsafe behavior. The self-acceptance of self-care calls the person to acknowledge her reality and to work positively within that reality. This is not to suggest that a person "accept" one's HIV status in the sense of adopting a fatalistic attitude. Rather, self-acceptance includes working within the limitations faced by and possibilities open to the person, and doing all that one can to maintain one's health holistically.

JUSTICE

In addition to our specific and unique relationships, we are part of a larger humanity, and the virtue of justice offers some insights into how we are to relate to one another generally. Justice reminds us that "we belong to humanity and are expected to respond to all its members in general, equally and impartially."[47] As the ethics of virtue asks us who we are, who we wish to become, and how do we get there, the virtue of justice specifically asks questions of us in light of the world community. What do human dignity and an embodied relational agency look like in our society and our world? What does our world look like as we see historical suffering and success? How are we envisioning, reflecting upon, and acting upon a vision of human flourishing for all? Justice engages our farsightedness, not to remove us from the near-neighbor but to bring us closer to 20/20 vision. Justice calls and challenges us to generativity for the "large haul." How we respond to this invitation depends on our understanding of and commitment to justice.

Much has been written about justice over the centuries. Thomas Aquinas defined the virtue of justice as "the constant and perpetual will to render to each one that which is his right."[48] Today a common understanding of justice is "giving to each one his or her due." But what criteria do we use to determine what one is "due"? Who determines the criteria? Is everyone with

HIV "due" pharmaceutical treatment? Who makes that determination? Pharmaceutical companies? Persons with HIV? Individual nations? The World Trade Organization? The United Nations? These are questions that are still debated today.

Charity is the foundation of the cardinal virtue of justice. The goal or telos of justice is love of God and love of neighbor. Whatever then is required by justice is already required by charity. What charity requires, however, may not be required of justice.[49]

Some contemporary thinkers are filling in the description and challenge of justice. Karen Lebacqz writes that "justice has to do with fulfilling the demands of relationships."[50] What are these demands, one might ask? Jeffrey Weeks states that "justice demands not only avoidance of unnecessary pain, but fostering care and responsibility for the other."[51] Here we see an attempt not only to "avoid evil" but also to "do good." This may account for some of the differences between minimal justice and maximum justice. Farley writes that "minimal justice, then, may have equality as its norm and full mutuality as its goal. Justice will be maximal as it approaches the ultimate goal of communion with each person, with all persons, and with God."[52] Justice at its maximum most closely mirrors love, and for Christians, Jesus is the exemplar of love and justice.

Catholic social thought has increasingly utilized need as the basic criterion for justice.[53] In their pastoral letter *Economic Justice for All*, the U.S. bishops articulated need as a primary reason for moral and social activity: "The fundamental moral criterion for all economic decisions, policies and institutions is this: they must be at the service of all people, especially the poor."[54] Cahill concurs when asserting, "In the Catholic tradition *justice* means precisely the association of persons in community according to relationships and structures that serve the good of all. Insofar as poverty and gender bias assist the spread of HIV, the recognition of the dignity of every woman and man is an essential precondition of diminishing infection."[55]

Justice then requires a recognition of the needs of persons and an awareness of the persons and structures that oppress as well as those that free. In 1971, the first modern congregational meeting of bishops to include a significant number of bishops from nonindustrialized or Third World countries produced *Justice in the World*, which proclaimed: "Even though it is not for us to elaborate a very profound analysis of the situation of the world, we have nevertheless been able to perceive the serious injustices which are building around the world of men a network of domination, oppression and abuses which stifle freedom and which keep the greater part of humanity from sharing in the building up and enjoyment of a more just and more fraternal world."[56] Lebacqz further writes that as justice "must include attention to the creation of goods, the participation of all in decision-making processes, and the rectification of historical injustices," we begin with a "recognition of structural problems of oppression."[57] We see in these descriptions advocacy for the person envisioned in our theological anthropology.

For further theological grounding of our understanding of justice, in addition to a Trinitarian model of a communion of equals in full mutuality,[58] Scripture remains an invaluable resource for grounding justice in the heart of the ministry of all persons: "Action on behalf of justice and participation in the transformation of the world fully appear to us as a constitutive dimension of the preaching of the Gospel, or, in other words, of the Church's mission for the redemption of the human race and its liberation from every oppressive situation."[59]

What does justice look like in our time of AIDS? Four markers of justice in terms of HIV/AIDS are (1) a critical knowledge of global structures and issues, (2) attentiveness to the needs of persons on the margins, (3) interior discipline, and (4) active, creative engagement.

Our first marker of justice, a critical knowledge of global structures and issues, takes both time and courage. In a frenetically busy society, justice requires that we take time to educate ourselves about the local and global world in which we live. A process of critical analysis is essential, and Catholic social teaching and the teachings of other concerned groups offer various models.[60] Social justice analysis always requires that as we learn about the realities of our world, we do so with questions about how institutions, policies, and practices affect the concrete situation of the poor and marginalized.

We will never know how U.S. domestic or foreign policy is affecting those on the margins unless we know something about the policy. This means that we not only read and listen to popular news media, but that we also have access to information that offers a more probing analysis of issues.[61] Modern technology brings more information from a variety of fronts than ever before. Internet sites on any number of specific justice issues abound. Although we need to carefully discriminate among information sources, many Catholic, ecumenical, and secular justice organizations and lobbying groups suggest web sites or journals with which to begin an investigation. For example, very fine international and accessible web sites with global and domestic HIV/AIDS information include www.caritasinternational.org and www.unaids.org. Moreover, since poverty is connected to HIV vulnerability, organizations such as Network and the Center for Concern have web sites related to these and other topics.

Most dioceses and many parishes also have Social Concerns committees. A key component of these committees is education. Education includes an assessment of both our domestic situation and our global influence in economics, politics, and culture. An understanding of our own nation is heightened by an understanding of situations in other nations and continents.

In this day and age, globalization and the influence of so many transnational institutions [e.g., the World Trade Organization and the World Bank] and corporations [e.g., McDonald's, Coca-Cola] require greater knowledge concerning how policies and laws are affecting the most vulnerable. As companies are assessed by organizations concerned with socially responsible investing, we must be willing to learn what our stocks are doing and how they affect the poor and most vulnerable. In an age where "spirituality and business" conferences abound, individual spiritual practices must include knowing how "just" our companies and investment practices are and reflecting upon who we are becoming through our association with them.

Courage is essential here. Whether an economy is in the midst of a "bear" or a "bull" market, it takes courage to look at our investments, policies, and practices while facing the poor, the marginalized, and persons with HIV/AIDS. Justice education is courageous because it has the potential to take us from our comfort zone to a less comfortable "growth" zone that will ask more of us. Critical global attentiveness may touch upon a fear of responsibility for what we know—yet it calls us to continue to learn. So while "the truth will set you free," our freedom exacts a price and requires courage. Justice demands the virtue of courage.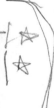

An awareness of the needs of those on the margins is our second marker of justice. Once we have information, it is important to find some experiential component to what we are learning. This means inviting people on the margins to meet us and our going to those on the margins. Here it is important to listen to persons with HIV or AIDS, and to those at risk for the virus. Important as well is listening to those who work with people on the margins, such as AIDS health care workers. Both groups have essential experiences, information, and even suggestions to share. Each group can nominally speak for the other, but neither can encompass the other. Justice requires that assessments of the AIDS situation and efforts to create solutions include those most affected by the disease. Justice for an embodied relational agent means that each person participates as fully as possible. A dimension of justice that becomes possible when we see, listen to, and hear people sharing their experiences is that we may find in their stories our own experiences of exclusion, our own "-isms." Perhaps we may realize that we have also excluded. An awareness of exclusion thus offers an opportunity to embrace.

A concrete demand of justice is that we somehow find opportunities to go to those on the margins. Inviting people to come speak to us in our comfort spaces is one way of learning about justice. However, the invitation to growth is also to go to the perhaps unfamiliar places where HIV/AIDS resides.[62] By doing so we acknowledge on yet another level the reality of people who share their stories. When we are invited in and are willing to enter and sit and hear the other's reality—the struggle, the pain, the successes—we can be more aware of the realities of those on the margins. Human dignity resides in these encounters, which are important dimensions of solidarity.[63] These experiences can be local or global, and the hope is that a community of believers will have in their midst enough diversity and openness to have all these elements.

A third marker of justice is that it requires the discipline of interiority. An interior groundedness is necessary if we are to be just people. To open our hearts, minds, and even resources to those whom we do not particularly know requires a deep sense of each person's innate human dignity and an attentiveness to the sacredness of all creation and our relatedness to all.[64] By focusing on relationships, we can also address the intention and disposition necessary for justice to be realized.

This interior discipline and disposition is a prayerful heart. Only a stance grounded in our deepest loves and relationships can bring us to the grace of risking what we have for the sake of another. A contemplative attentiveness and engagement can bring us to the brink of minimal and maximum justice and offer us the grace for a next step. Although both minimal and maximum justice may entail sacrifice, reflective living can move us to a love that can sacrifice. The Paschal mystery is again evident in works of justice, for it was Jesus' love that led him to the cross. In St. Paul's writings we see that the "death and resurrection of Jesus Christ is the manifestation of the work of God's justice in an unjust world. As noted of the Servant in the Old Testament, Jesus is the just one who suffers innocently at the hands of unjust people but, in the process conquers them (Col 2:15) and makes humans reconciled to God's justice (2 Cor. 5:21)."[65]

Interior discipline grounds us so that we have the capacity for the "long haul" and the "large haul." Without an interior rootedness, we can become overwhelmed or burned out as we respond to the challenge of HIV/AIDS.[66] Persons may have experiences that open their eyes to the suffering of others, and compassion moves them to find ways to improve the situation. Jumping in to do what can be done is important. However, what happens as the person realizes that the situation in Africa continues to deteriorate, or that only small improvements are being made while larger ones are needed? Will the person stay committed or become frustrated and lose heart? What will be the well of wisdom into which the jar of discernment will dip? It is what lies deepest within us, the source of hope within us as well as outside of us, that keeps us going. Prayer grounds us so that we do not burn out or drown in the suffering, but instead have the strength to persevere. When we have firmly rooted companions on this journey, justice flourishes beyond any one lifetime. This prayerful rootedness is the flame that keeps the spark alive. It is our strength.

Creative, active engagement is the fourth marker of justice. People often think of justice solely in terms of action, yet action requires the other three indicators in order for us to determine the appropriate course of action. Depending on the situation, there may be a variety of options and actions, and many of them for good. However, justice does ultimately demand some form of active engagement.

The "law of graduality" considers justice a growth process. Action on behalf of justice can evolve from just preventing harm to doing good, for the good of each and all.[67] According to Burggraeve's minimum for sexual ethics as the "no harm principle," justice in the case of casual sex minimally requires condom use to assist with HIV prevention for both persons. Similarly for a female sex worker, justice minimally requires clients to use condoms to prevent HIV and to protect her as she earns money to provide for herself and her family. Justice on a larger scale seeks out alternative sources of income for women so that their human dignity need not be compromised by the sale of their bodies.

The creative component of justice includes finding new ways to approach problems. Drugs for treating HIV/AIDS patients have been very expensive, and this limits access to the populations who can afford treatment. Pharmaceutical companies control access to drugs by controlling the price demanded for them. Industrialized countries were among the few groups able to absorb these costs. However, when a company in India announced that it could manufacture generic drugs for a fraction of the cost of competitors, the pharmaceutical industry was sent spinning, and poor countries found a hopeful voice for their cause. At the same time, the larger worldwide public, galvanized by their shock and anger at the pharmaceutical industry, challenged what they perceived as greed and pressured the industry into taking some responsibility for the human community in need. The drug companies felt the great public outrage. A factor that further pressured companies to make their drugs more accessible was Brazil's assertion through example that, contrary to public opinion, the poor and marginalized were able to follow the extensive regimen required for drug treatment to be effective.[68] Here we see justice galvanized through a number of areas, through both individual action and systemic challenge. Companies subsequently lowered their prices.[69] Access to drug treatment and problems related to distribution continue to offer invitations for creative activity.

We must now ask how we make determinations when there are competing claims for justice, or even among the virtues. How do we make these determinations? Keenan reminds us that "justice rests on impartiality and universality," and that "fidelity rests on partiality and particularity."[70] What, then, do we do when partial and impartial claims compete, as they invariably can and do? What happens when fidelity is in tension with justice? What if self-care makes the claim that my need at this moment is greater than the need of the other I do not know? For answers to these questions we consider prudence, our final virtue.

PRUDENCE: TOWARD A MORALLY CREATIVE IMAGINATION

Because fidelity, self-care, and justice are not ethically prior to or superior to one another, the virtue of prudence is needed to determine the way one is to live. Aquinas invokes Aristotle's claim that prudence is "right reason about things to be done."[71] This right moral reasoning includes not only one's decision-making, but indeed the whole of one's life. As a virtue it considers not simply what we do, but more importantly, who we will become: "Prudence is of good counsel about matters regarding man's entire life and the end of human life."[72] Yves R. Simon reminds us that when a difficult decision is made, prudence both weighs the claims of the other virtues and flows out of our basic dispositions and who we are at a given point in time.[73] Prudence has a privileged place among the cardinal virtues, for it "recognizes the ends to which a person is naturally inclined, it establishes the agenda by which one can pursue those ends, it directs the agent's own performance of the pursued activity, and, finally, it measures the rightness of the actions taken."[74] In discerning the "good life," prudence is marked by the following markers and tasks: (1) to pursue the ends to which the person is naturally inclined; (2) to integrate the other cardinal virtues; (3) to engage the moral imagination; and (4) to establish a moral agenda for a person growing in virtue.

Prudence presumes a vision and pursues an end. While prudence does not determine the last end of each virtue, it articulates all the proximate ends, and pursues those of even the last end. Aquinas and others see practical or right moral reason as a capacity of most persons.[75] For Aquinas "the proper end of each moral virtue consists precisely in conformity with right reason."[76] One could, then, attain natural ends, such as those of natural law, with prudence. However, the ultimate end or telos that Christians seek by faith is union with God in love. Charity is needed for prudence to be disposed to this end.[77] Though both are significant, the task of prudence in light of charity is greater than that without charity as the end.

For us today this means that prudence pursues the ends that we most value. If what we value most is to do good and avoid evil, prudence works with that vision. If our greatest goal is to love God, neighbor, and ourselves, then that is the end for which prudence strives. Here it is important to again realize that ends can be developmental as well as multidimensional. If living an option for the poor and marginalized is my goal, prudence will pursue that. However, internal tensions can arise when prudence asks whether something is a claim of justice or of self-care. Knowing what our ends actually are helps us to be honest with ourselves and to mediate the internal conflicts that can occur when we name one goal and really seek another. A clear end allows our whole, embodied, relational agency to strive for this actuality, even as we may be any number of places on the road. An end offers a context for the content of the virtues.

Prudence has as its second task to integrate the other cardinal virtues into one's life and life decisions. On its own, prudence lacks the content necessary for determining the kind of life I will live. The other three cardinal virtues provide the content from which a prudential, integrated life is constructed. Though the other three virtues have no priority over one another, prudence depends on the other cardinal virtues to offer insights about particular, general, and unique relationships. When a conflict occurs, as it often does among relationships and values, prudence determines which is the greater claim.[78] When claims conflict, prudence probes what each of the other cardinal virtues offers in terms of wisdom and experience. Here, too, Simon reminds us that we must take into consideration that we will not possess all virtues to the same degree.[79] Questions are again asked of our relationships and of the claims they have on us. When a decision is made, prudence engages in a fully embodied—emotional, spiritual, intellectual, physical—discernment.

Active, relational, and intentionally reflective lives provide content for our decisions. Prudence is the fruit of who we are at a given point in time as embodied relational agents. Sometimes decisions are quick—such as running into the street to pull a child out of the way of an approaching car, or offering a spontaneous donation after hearing a moving presentation on impoverished conditions in Appalachia. Some decisions are slowly weighed and deliberated, such as where I will invest my time or how I will invest my fiscal resources. However, these decisions are all the fruit of who we are becoming and seeking to be. We seek to live out our desires, and the practice of virtues offers solid material from which prudence can direct us to our greatest desires.

Prudence, the integration of our virtues to the end we seek, takes time. Prudence must also be practiced so that as more life experiences, insights, and desires are internalized and integrated, a spiral of prudence emerges that influences even the smaller parts of one's life.

Although it is not often associated with prudence, a third marker of this virtue is moral imagination.[80] We all have a moral imagination through which we work out our vision of human flourishing.[81] The "Christian" moral imagination refers to some of the resources our Christian faith experience and tradition offer us as we strive to live so that all humans flourish. This is the imagination we engage in the situation of HIV/AIDS.[82]

In light of the pandemic of AIDS, full human flourishing requires that we see beyond "the surface" of facts around us to possibilities that can be realized around us. To see AIDS and imagine only further and future devastation of human life in its physical, economic, and social manifestations is one way of envisioning the human. However, Christianity and the moral imagination flowing out of that point of view offer a different horizon of expectations and, I contend, ensuing actions. The Christian imagination is rooted in the real but imagines more than what is seen, because, as mentioned earlier in this chapter, for Christians the horizon of expectations is rooted in hope.

Philip Keane describes imagination as "the basic process by which we draw together the concrete and the universal elements of our human experience . . . a playful suspension of judgment leading us toward a more appropriate grasp of reality."[83] This "playful suspension" is not one of reality but of judgment about the reality. Imagination here is not fantasy, which makes up or creates an image to avoid or escape reality. Imagination instead takes various experiences and realities and places them in a context, an "intelligible landscape."[84] William F. Lynch sees imagination as remaking reality and connects imagination quite directly with hope. Lynch reminds us:

> one of the permanent meanings of imagination has been that it is the gift that envisions what cannot yet be seen, the gift that constantly proposes to itself that the boundaries of the possible are wider than they seem. Imagination, if it is in prison and has tried every exit, does not panic or move into apathy but sits down to try to envision another way out. It is always slow to admit that all the facts are in, that all the doors have been tried, and that it is defeated. It is not so much that it has vision as that it is able to wait, to wait for a moment of vision which is not yet there, for a door that is not yet locked. It is not overcome by the absoluteness of the present moment.[85]

So far we see that the engagement of the imagination in our moral life offers three important insights. First, it is a whole, embodied experience, in which all of the senses are engaged. Second, the moral imagination is a point of view from which we creatively and constructively interact with reality. Third, the moral imagination is where we work out our vision of human flourishing. A fourth element to be linked more specifically to the Christian moral imagination is the use of analogy, through which we build the bridge from our contemporary experiences and our faith tradition, including our Scripture, to prudential action.

Our capacity for analogy helps us connect and integrate elements of our tradition with our experiences and information about our contemporary world.[86] The analogical imagination is a lens through which we see in order to distill the essential insights from our faith and apply them to our lives and world around us. Scripture and tradition give us a sense of the horizon of our expectations. In this way we are not held to "what Jesus would do" in a situation, but we are invited to live "what Jesus is doing now through me" as an incarnation. The imagination is helpful, for as Jesus remains the "concrete universal of Christian ethics, the paradigm that normatively guides Christian living," we are able to move analogically from Jesus' story to discovering how to move daily toward a reality reflective of the Reign of God.[87]

The ability to draw analogy offers us a way in which to reflect on the story of the leper who was cured by Jesus (Mt 8:1–4). This story is no longer limited to lepers, but includes all who are deemed outcasts by society. Jesus' response is not only to touch, but to heal with his touch. Jesus welcomed the outcasts and invited them back to the community. We, too, are called to welcome back into our churches and communities modern-day lepers on our margins, persons with HIV/AIDS. Our sense of community must welcome all. The analogical imagination does not claim that we yet have a cure for AIDS, but it offers us a vision for our response to persons with AIDS. Through the imagination we see more than the illness; we see the person and we find ways to invite him or her into the community. The way we invite our communities to respond to the reality of AIDS is part of this embodied relational engagement. This is also true in terms of how we must imagine structures and institutions necessary for constructively dealing with HIV/AIDS (e.g., pharmaceutical companies; government research funds; NGOs; and diocesan, national, and international church initiatives).

The fourth marker of prudence is that it establishes a moral agenda for people and for society. A constructively critical attitude is necessary, for we must cultivate a "capacity for self-criticism" as we examine both the world around us and ourselves in light of the cardinal virtues.[88] Our decisions and deliberations tell us both where we have grown and where growth is still necessary. Our practices are both internal and external indicators of who we are becoming. Who we are becoming is also known through the ends we seek and pursue. Both ends and means, in a reflectively active life, continue to spiral more deeply toward our greatest desires and more fully toward the loves we pursue.

A moral agenda is a communal issue, for as a community and society, we are also constantly "becoming." We must together ask whether our deliberations and acts as a Christian community and as a nation coincide with or collide with what we claim as our greatest values. Prudence expects such participation and dialogue.

The virtues truly bring our theological anthropology to life. They offer form for the content, and we can see how our Christian tradition continually engages and animates a vision of life that flows through the virtues. In the midst of a world struggling with HIV/AIDS, we will now focus more directly on Christian spirituality as a grounding for our ethics and an ethics to awaken the Christian community to respond to the AIDS crisis. We turn to Christian discipleship in our next chapter.

QUESTIONS FOR REFLECTION AND DISCUSSION

1. Which virtue do you find most compelling? Why?
2. If you were to add an additional virtue needed for this time of AIDS, what would it be? Explain.
3. What practices and attitudes have you found that cultivate the virtues mentioned in this chapter (hope, fidelity, self-care, justice, and prudence)?
4. When have you engaged your moral imagination? What happened?

CHAPTER 5

Discipleship:
The Response of Spirituality and
Morality in an Age of AIDS

As we approach discipleship in an age of AIDS, we mindfully locate our discussion within the Christian tradition because of the named and shared experience of God expressing love for us, and because of our desire to respond in turn to God's love through a life of love. Our experience of God helps us decide on a common starting point for our being and doing. This common starting point calls the entire Christian community to respond to the situation of AIDS in light of what we value most and believe. Though it does not mandate *how* we respond, it does mandate *that* we respond. The call to us as Christians is both personal and communal, and thus our response to HIV/AIDS today must be on both levels.

we must respond...

personal & communal

In this chapter, the integrated sense of Christian spirituality and morality that is needed for the church community to adequately respond to HIV/AIDS is defined and developed within the context of discipleship. Following this, some of the contemporary obstacles to discipleship are discussed.

INTEGRATING CHRISTIAN SPIRITUALITY
AND CHRISTIAN MORALITY

Forty years ago, the Church began to appreciate again the need to integrate spirituality and morality in the Christian life. Before that time, from the sixteenth century until about 1960, moral theology separated the moral life from the spiritual or ascetic life.[1] During the last forty years, the call by moral theology to reintegrate spirituality and morality has often been within the context of discipleship. One of the first theologians to call for such an integration was Fritz Tillman, whose work *The Master Calls: A Handbook of Christian Living* "integrated a Scripturally-based ethics into a discipleship model that was rooted in ascetical theology."[2] Shortly after this, Bernard

Häring's work *The Law of Christ* was published, which followed an *imitatio Christi* model for discipleship ethics.[3] Subsequently, many other moral theologians have written within a discipleship context, including, recently, William Spohn, Richard Gula, and Timothy O'Connell.[4]

As Christians we identify ourselves as followers of Jesus Christ. Discipleship is about a way of life as a follower of Jesus, the initiator of the call to each of us to follow him. This way of life is fed and nourished by our spirituality and flows into the life we live and into the world around us. The call to integrate spirituality and morality within the context of discipleship is an essential viewpoint from which to consider living in the world. It is as disciples that we respond to AIDS, on both an individual and a communal scale. Indeed, there is a particular claim on the Christian community because of this integrated way of living spiritually and morally.

Christian spirituality and Christian morality, although distinct disciplines, are continually integrating with and interpenetrating one another.

Spirituality is first of all about a way of life that seeks to reflect and embody what gives ultimate meaning and value to life for a person.[5] As such, everyone has a spirituality. Christian spirituality is a Christ-centered way of life that considers God to be the greatest love and desire.

Although there are certainly many definitions of Christian spirituality, recently theologians have described it in a way that is inclusive of the moral life. David Lonsdale describes Christian spirituality as "the attempt to give an orientation to the whole of one's daily living under the influence of the Spirit of Christ and the gospel."[6] Philip Sheldrake writes that "In Christian terms, 'spirituality' concerns how people subjectively appropriate traditional beliefs about God, the human person, creation, and their interrelationship, and then express these in worship, basic values and lifestyle. Thus, spirituality is the whole of human life viewed in terms of a conscious relationship with God, in Jesus Christ, through the indwelling of the Spirit and within the community of believers."[7] Richard Gula's description highlights the integration of spirituality and morality for discipleship. Gula writes that Christian spirituality is "a way of discipleship involving a personal relationship with Jesus under the power of the Holy Spirit working in and through the community of believers to bring about a world marked by justice and peace."[8]

Similarly, Christian morality, although still a separate discipline, is increasingly described in connection with the spiritual life. Morality concerns the way we live in the world today as followers of Jesus. For a long time morality was predominantly connected with acts, with doing the "right" thing and following norms and rules. Moral formation now includes the growth and development of character through practices, dispositions, and acts. Mark O'Keefe describes the moral life as "fundamentally a life of grateful response to God's offer of relationship in Christ. God offers a share in the divine life itself, a share in God's own holiness. The Christian life is a life of discipleship, following Jesus, that involves becoming morally good as the foundation to attaining, by God's grace, the holiness to which God invites us."[9]

Discipleship based in spirituality finds itself flourishing in morality. Spirituality nourishes the moral life, and in so doing animates and shapes morality. As disciples we are incorporated into a community that also seeks to follow Jesus. As we are animated and seek to follow Jesus in this way, we find ourselves asking how we can serve this world in which we live. That is *the* moral question because it puts our spirituality into moral expression. A spirituality of discipleship finds its expression in morality, in moral ways of living. Richard Gula perhaps expresses best the distinction and interconnection between spirituality and morality in the disciple's life. Gula writes,

> Spirituality, with its array of practices, nourishes the moral life at its very roots by deepening our awareness of being loved and by energizing our commitment to living in a way that makes this love a real, transforming presence in the world. Spirituality is the wellspring of the moral life. That is to say that morality arises from, rather than generates, spirituality. The moral journey begins in that spiritual space where we accept God's love for us and awaken to responsibility for promoting the well-being of persons and the community in harmony with the environment. In this way, morality reveals one's spirituality.[10]

This spiritual and moral journey is the way of discipleship.

SIX ELEMENTS OF DISCIPLESHIP

With these descriptions as helpful starting points, I will focus on six elements of discipleship which mark an integrated Christian spiritual and moral life essential for a positive response to AIDS today.[11] They are necessary if the Christian community is to offer a life-promoting response in the midst of the AIDS pandemic.

1. *Christian discipleship as a way of life begins with God expressing love for us.*[12]

Seeking God as our greatest love and desire is possible because we believe that God first loved us. God is the source of all love. Although it is impossible to name all the ways that God's love reaches out to us, the love of God is not some abstract notion. There is some way in which we experience the love of God in our lives. We often first come to know the love of God from people who love us. In a very real way, God becomes present to us through the love and care of other people.[13] We may be touched by God's love in the beauty we experience in nature or in a symphony. We may encounter deep joy in solitude or in being with others. There are limitless possibilities for the experience of God's love. Yet at the core of Christian spirituality there is a personal experience of God reaching out to us in love, and of our acceptance of that love.[14]

2. Our response to God's love is a way of life.

Once we receive this love, even a hint of it, we seek also to respond in love, through all the events of our lives. The fire that burns and grows within us seeks outward expression. This love is a fire that both illuminates and gives us a sense of the goodness of all creation. This outward expression is found in the way we love and care for others and for the earth. Our response to God's love is our way of relating to God, to others, and to ourselves.[15] We seek greater depths of love of God and love of neighbor. We continually grow in our openness to receiving and responding to love.

3. Christian discipleship as a way of life is an expression of one's faith and love.

Our lived spirituality is an expression of what we believe about God, Jesus, and the Holy Spirit. Christians believe in a personal, loving God who shared life with us and who revealed Godself to us through Jesus Christ. Jesus Christ continues to be revealed to us through the Holy Spirit working in and through the community of believers. Disciples of Jesus today have had a personal encounter with Jesus Christ and now seek to live in his same spirit. Each generation encounters the message, challenge, and invitation of Jesus' life anew, and how we respond is an expression of where we are in integrating what we most deeply believe.[16] Although our faith is a gift, it is a gift that must be nurtured and developed over time.[17]

4. Discipleship is a way of life lived as a member of a community of believers.

Christians are incorporated into a community that professes belief in God, Jesus Christ, and the Holy Spirit and that seeks to love in response to the God who first loved us. Our spirituality is in some way shaped by this community at the same time that we also shape the community. As community members, our response to God, though always personal, also has communal dimensions. Community reminds us of our inherently relational nature and values the gifts of each person. The community is a dynamic, Spirit-led body that seeks to respond to God's gift of love through worship and service. As a lens through which we see God acting in our midst, community calls us to personal, communal, and societal transformation.

Although moral theology has at times been restricted to the individual and even private sphere, Catholic spirituality and its social tradition remind moral theology of the social agenda for action. In recent years one of morality's contributions is that it has helped us not only understand the individual as historical and unique, but also recognize our "embeddedness in unjust structures and of our responsibility for the environment in which we live and in which others are yet to live . . . Morality . . . has freed people to be creative and imaginative."[18] Structural transformation for the common good is an essential part of the moral agenda in the world today. In our earlier discussion of justice we saw both Catholic social teaching and the Gospels cited to support change for the benefit of all. We must also not miss the fact that the communities and groups calling for structural change are usually those who are suffering. Those in positions of structural power do not often desire change. These include political, economic, and ecclesial institutions and their leaders.

The commitment of the community of disciples is to bring about the Reign of God in justice and peace for all people. Our call extends beyond those we know to all persons, and particularly to those in need. How we do all this leads us to our next point.

5. *Christian discipleship as a way of life requires spiritual exercises and practices.*

Practices and exercises are meant to draw us closer to God, to our neighbor, and to ourselves. Practices, both personal and communal, keep us attentive to and connected to the Source of love in our lives. They are meant to draw us closer to God, to those we love, to our neighbors near and far, and to ourselves. They also keep us open to responding in love. Our love for one another, whether through fidelity to the one we know or through justice to the neighbor we do not know, grows and is sustained by our practices.

The life and message of Jesus is about love, and simultaneously it is about the cost of love, which can include suffering. We cannot bear the price of love and encounter suffering without connection to the fire of love within us, which is God. This requires practices that keep us close to the pulse of our ultimate values and desires. Only then will we dare to hear the pulse of the other in need and respond to that need.

Although there are many ways to practice Christian spirituality, they are all forms of prayer. They are ways of opening ourselves to an encounter with the divine around us, in us, and in one another. As such, prayer can be personal or communal. There are also many forms of prayer, and I briefly mention two: reading Scripture and participating in liturgy. As discipleship is about following Jesus, a central source from which we can learn about Jesus is Scripture. Sandra Schneiders reminds us that we read Scripture for *transformation* rather than information.[19] The analogical imagination is again relevant, for "the story of Jesus is a *paradigm*, a normative pattern or exemplar that can be creatively applied in different circumstances."[20] Jesus' life and teachings are normative for our lives as disciples.[21] The story of Jesus of Nazareth shapes our way of life, not only for imitation but also as inspiration, guidance, and direction for our way of encountering the world around us. Scripture invites both a personal and communal engagement, and time for each is important for sustaining the person and the community.

Liturgy is a communal form of worship. We gather to connect with God in all parts of our lives, offering praise, petition, and thanksgiving. Liturgy personally and communally connects us to and reminds us of the collective vision and mission we have as disciples. The message, challenge, and invitation of Jesus' life are fresh for each generation as we encounter him. How we respond is an expression of how we integrate what we most deeply believe.

6. *Christian discipleship as a way of life requires moral praxis.*

A way of life that keeps us connected to God's love and that helps us deepen our love for all contains a profound and abiding sense of the beauty and sacredness of all people. It is just such experiences of love and goodness which galvanize efforts to bring about a world "marked by justice and peace."[22] Christian spirituality and morality require that we attend to those suffering on the margins of society. When we meet people on the margins, when we encounter suffering on the margins, or when we see structural injustice, these are such jarring experiences that we respond with resistance to suffering by offering assistance to those who suffer.

There are resources available to us as we encounter our world and offer a response. Conscience formation and discernment are necessary in all areas of our lives.[23] Anne Patrick describes the process of discernment well: "Christian ethics draws from the wisdom of the religious tradition as well as that of secular disciplines, including philosophy and the sciences, to provide data about the likely effects of various choices as well as clarity about ways of discerning value and making moral judgments."[24] Our encounter with our God and the world around us is a fully embodied response, engaging all of us individually and communally.

A particular response to suffering on the margins is denoted by the term *praxis*. Rebecca S. Chopp writes that praxis signifies "intentional social activity and the need for emancipatory transformation."[25] The primacy of praxis in recent years is partly the result of greater acknowledgment of and attention to structural crises such as poverty, the Holocaust, and various social injustices such as sexism and racism.[26] The AIDS crisis is perhaps one of the newer crises to evoke a similar cry for social transformation. Just as theological anthropology and the virtues are components of a spirituality for this age of AIDS, praxis is a necessary partner to those efforts. Praxis "serves to speak of a new way of envisioning spirituality and theology, of viewing human subjects and history, of configuring Christian faith and symbols, and of speaking to the crisis of structural and psychic suffering in the contemporary situation."[27]

This praxis is carried out not only by individuals but also very much by communities. The community is a lens through which we see God acting in our midst, calling us and society to change. The spiritual life for us includes praxis as "the embodied activity of Christian faith and its communal character in transforming situations and experiences of suffering into those of freedom."[28] To bring about the Reign of God in justice and peace for all people is a commitment of the community.

By way of summary, then, we see that these six elements of Christian discipleship are components of a call and a response to a personal and loving God. Spirituality and morality are inseparable from one another in the life of a disciple. Patrick asserts: "There can be no impenetrable boundaries between the disciplines of spiritual theology and Christian ethics, for both concern the vision of what human well-being and authentic discipleship involve. Spirituality supplies the vision and the motivation, the context within which ethics matters . . . The relationship between these two theological disciplines is reciprocal and complementary, and both are accountable to the same biblical norm that has been modeled so definitively in Jesus: 'This is what Yahweh asks of you, only this: to act justly, to love tenderly, and to walk humbly with your God' (Mic 6: 8)."[29]

OBSTACLES TO DISCIPLESHIP

In the preceding section we discussed some of the essential components of Christian discipleship. In this section we turn to some of the obstacles to a life of discipleship.

If discipleship is such an integrating task and life, why doesn't the world look better than it does? Why is the global Christian community not responding more effectively to HIV/AIDS? The answers to these questions are complicated. Vincent Macnamara states that we must want to be moral, and that spiritual growth is about growing in sensitivity to the moral strands of our experiences. It is a process of conversion.[30] Once we desire to be moral, we must take responsibility for discovering how we are to specifically express this desire. And the truth we may hear within us and around us may not be easy.[31] There is a cost to discipleship; it is not "cheap grace."[32]

There are many obstacles to discipleship in our time that hinder and stall efforts to address the AIDS crisis; a brief description of just four of these challenges follows: (1) frenetic activity, (2) contextual communities resisting diversity, (3) risk aversion/fear, and (4) paralysis. These are crucial challenges to address in the United States and in many other industrialized nations.

A great obstacle to discipleship in our culture is frenetic activity. We are busy with many things, and we must ask what drives and grounds our usually well-meaning busyness. We seek more of everything—more experiences, more stimulation, more access to resources, more relationships. However, when we are trying to respond to the suffering around us, frenetic activity denies us the grounding we need to address suffering sufficiently. Frenzied busyness prevents us from knowing the other with any depth. Experiences pile up one after the other, and the nature of our lives prevents us from finding the depth in those experiences. Running from one activity to another, even when the activities are worthwhile, can result in a kind of moral numbness. When we do not take time to pause and reflect on our experiences and our relationships, their depth of meaning gets lost. Even setting directions for the work of justice is problematic if we do not take the time to determine the foundations that are to be questioned (e.g., foundational causes of AIDS). And ultimately, our level of commitment and a loving embodied response to the other become muted when they are not grounded. A collection of experiences without grounding in our ultimate meaning (God) stalls at some point.

When we are excessively busy it is difficult for mind and heart and body to respond in an integrated way. Thus, the busyness of our lives can keep us from connecting as fully embodied people to other people.

We must vigilantly ask what this hectic activity is really about. Does my activity speak to what gives my life meaning? Is it a matter of greed—accumulating experiences, money, material possessions, etc.? Are we so busy in ministry because we consider ourselves to be the only people who can meet needs? Are we trying to avoid "dealing" with ourselves? What are my experiences of giving and receiving love in the midst of all this activity? Discipleship is about the "long haul," a vision beyond even our own lifetimes. Constant activity, though perhaps well intended, does not allow space for the spiritual life to flow through the moral life for the long haul.

A second obstacle to discipleship is the contextual community that resists diversity. We naturally wish to live, worship, and work with and relate to those with whom we are most comfortable. Often "comfortable" means "those most like us." Contextual communities that resist diversity may be found in our churches, our neighborhoods, our workplaces, our religious communities, our friendships. These communities may be uncomfortable welcoming or even engaging with others who are significantly different from themselves. The differences may be related to gender, race, education, lifestyle, economics, politics, geography, or religion.

Communities can become so contextual that they are isolated from other communities, particularly the marginalized. Bringing in the voices of the refugee, the gay, the poor, the divorced, and the woman remains an uncommon experience in many churches and parishes. Our parish communities sometimes think of the "other" as stranger and forget that Jesus welcomed all to the table, all to the community. Even when some of these voices are included, the contextual community remains intact if these new voices are seen solely as objects of concern and not also as agents who offer something to the community with which they engage. A community without diversity is an impoverished community.

A false sense of security is engendered in communities that avoid the difficult questions that emerge from listening and mutually engaging persons on the margins. Another illusion, perhaps, is that our lives will be less complicated if we remain in our comfortable communities. A final illusion might be that we need not face our own brokenness when our communities offer the fantasy that "God is in heaven and all is right with the world." Communities with such illusions eventually decrease in size, for few people live life without the challenge of suffering and loss.

A third obstacle to discipleship is risk aversion. As a society, the United States is increasingly risk averse. We resist paying a price for our faith or our loves. Our Gospel quite directly offers a Jesus of Nazareth who not only lived in love and offered healing, but who also spoke truths that were difficult to hear and who ultimately paid with his life for the message he lived and preached. When we are fearful of losing what we have, the needs of the other become secondary. We forget that our faith tradition calls us to share time, talents, and treasure; to sacrifice; and to work together for justice and peace for all people. We may verbally agree to these principles, but the real-life possibility carries frightening implications.

Exploring the dynamic dimension of our tradition as we read and respond to the "signs of the times" is a particular area of risk aversion in our Church today. In some arenas, critical and creative fidelity is deemed suspicious at best and heretical at worst. Although there is agreement that the Church should be at the center of the tradition, fear arises when the Church moves us to the growing edges of the tradition. The prophetic dimension of the Church is denied when we fear to reexamine teachings in light of history, new information, and the experiences of the people of God. The prophetic dimension of the Church is denied when mandates replace love and when the suffering of people is not heard by those who have ears to hear and resources with which to respond. For example, in the case of HIV/AIDS, discussion of topics such as prophylactics and gender inequalities is discouraged in some parts of the Church. When such discussions are muted, the Church's credibility also diminishes. If we are to be able to risk, something greater than what we have must call us.

One expression of risk aversion is paralysis. The magnitude of the problems and the suffering of the world around us are overwhelming. How do I respond to almost 40 million people with HIV/AIDS? How do we as a faith community respond? Even when we do find ways to directly respond, we quickly realize that there are social and structural components of HIV/AIDS, and these can be overwhelming too. Responsibility for structural injustice is deemed the purview of a privileged, powerful few, and many of us feel we have no influence over government budgets or multinational corporations' policies. The immense dimensions of the issues may lead to paralysis. We may not know where to begin to address these issues, and we sense that our own resources are not sufficient. We may feel alone in trying to effect the necessary change on a global scale. We forget that most action begins on a local rather than a global scale. We forget to seek out others who share our concerns. We forget the power of communal discernment and action. When we forget, despair, that deep sense that nothing can be done and that there is no hope for the future, may set in. And therefore we may do nothing.

These are but a few of the major obstacles to Christian discipleship and to AIDS efforts today. They are significant challenges for a Christian spiritual and moral life, but an integrated life does offer a response. In Chapter 6 we turn to one such response.

QUESTIONS FOR REFLECTION AND DISCUSSION

1. Explain the connection between spirituality and morality.
2. What elements of discipleship do you find most challenging?
3. Which obstacles to discipleship in an age of AIDS do you notice in yourself? Do you notice any obstacles in your local faith community or church? How might these be addressed?
4. What people, organizations, or groups offer you a good example of an integrated spiritual and moral life? What do you think sustains this way of living? Is it possible to ask the person or a member of the organization?

CHAPTER 6

Memory, Narrative, and Solidarity

Johann Metz's key categories of memory, narrative, and solidarity offer a strategy for addressing the challenges of discipleship and, consequently, HIV/AIDS prevention and treatment efforts.[1]

Three important ways to keep the disciple open to the Gospel and open to the world as it really is, are to look at how and what we remember and why; which narratives we tell and why; and how and to whom we respond in solidarity. Our discussion of memory, narrative, and solidarity is rooted in the efforts of our preceding chapters. Our memories, narratives, and efforts at solidarity flow out of our vision of what it is to be human in our context today, out of how this humanity is brought to life, and out of the spirit that animates and directs our living and loving.

MEMORY

Memory is our capacity and ability to recall, to remember a past event, to bring something of history into our present reality.[2] We each have memories, and they fall anywhere along the spectrum from wonderful to painful. Our memories include experiences of loving and of failing to love, of being loved and of being rejected, of growth and regression, and of success and of failure. Our memories of shared experiences are also in some sense unique to each of us. For example, two siblings may attend a wedding and yet have two very different experiences of it.

We have collective memories as well, and these too have common denominators and distinctions. For example, in an era of instantaneous and mass communication, the hijacking and crashing of four planes on September 11, 2001 was in many ways a global experience. The image of the plane crashes and devastation could be the same for all, yet the memory had different connotations, depending on the perspective of the person and community. Our memories are embodied, and they are imbued with our history, beliefs, emotions, knowledge, and perspective on life.

Over thirty years ago Johann Baptist Metz began to speak of "dangerous memories," which Ashley describes as "memories which continually disrupt the smooth processes of reason, and in so disrupting, save it from a catastrophic self-absorption."[3] The understanding of memory that grounds Metz's approach to Christianity is rooted in his own experiences and memories. Two dangerously disruptive memories marked his life: (1) the experience of seeing his whole company wiped out when he was a conscripted sixteen-year-old soldier in Hitler's army and (2) the experience of a theology which never faced the Holocaust. For Metz, dangerous memories are rooted in history and society, and since histories are often written from the perspective of the winners, they do not necessarily recognize the impact of suffering on those who are not "winners."

Metz reminds us not to lose the truth of history as we seek to see the God of history at work in history. This is a challenge for our individual and collective memories. In terms of our painful memories of suffering in history, the challenge is not to try to simply or preemptively "make peace" with the memories, but instead to bring those memories to God with all the questions and pain that they encompass. Metz challenges us to consider "what would happen if one took this sort of remembrance not to the psychologist but into the Church? And if one did not allow oneself to be talked out of such unreconciled memories even by theology, but rather wanted to have faith with them and, with them, speak about God?"[4] Metz forces us to remember when love did not prevail, and to bring all this to our God and into our Church.

Unlike the Holocaust, HIV/AIDS is still a present event. With a known history of over twenty years, AIDS is both a memory of the past and an ongoing event. AIDS is our common history and our common present. Because it is a present event, HIV/AIDS affords us opportunities to intervene in the midst of the pandemic to halt the devastation. Whether a personal memory or not, with so many affected worldwide, HIV/AIDS is a collective memory of the global community. Memory entails remembering the victims of history who have suffered and died as well as those who are currently suffering. Neither the dead nor the living are forgotten. Discipleship today, in love, worship, and service, must be lived as we face all that is associated with HIV/AIDS. Such living takes a tremendous amount of courage.

We are able to live as disciples and face AIDS because as Christians we have a second set of dangerous memories. The history of our faith contains dangerous memories of scripture. As Christians we know our paradigmatic memory to be the life, death, and resurrection of Jesus Christ.[5] This memory is dangerous for at least three reasons. The first is that we are forced to stop at the cross. Ela writes that "the struggles of our people bring the memory of the Crucified One right into our own life and times."[6] Jesus' entire life opens us up to the suffering of others as well as to our own suffering. The second reason is that we have hope in the resurrection, in new life that results from a love that is stronger than the threat of death or even of death itself. The memory of the resurrection does not negate or even ultimately answer suffering, but it is a hopeful, lived expectation of a future that is to come. This is the future toward which we work. We celebrate these dangerous memories of our faith tradition in our liturgical life, for both cross and resurrection are present as we recount Jesus' life. Thus a third reason these are dangerous memories is that they include us in the entire paschal mystery. As Oduyoye notes, "We cannot assign the cross to half of humanity and the resurrection to the other half. Our theology of the cross and resurrection must remain together."[7] And we can do so precisely because we have a hope in which to ground our courage.

Memory requires that our frenetic activity stop long enough for us to see those outside of ourselves who are suffering. A context of faith can bring us to a view of people's lives in history that is broader than our own. At the same time, memory helps us to locate our struggles and suffering at the cross and to continue to bring these to God, even in "soundless cries."[8] Our hope for ourselves and for others is in a God who offers a narrative that goes beyond death, and in a community that strives to live that hopeful message on a daily basis.

Memories are a powerful resource for us as disciples. What we remember is a crucial tool for responding to the world around us. What, then, are we to do with these memories, and what of the memories of those whose experiences are different from ours? For this we turn to narratives.

NARRATIVE

Narratives are vehicles of communication, a telling of our memory as its meaning continues to evolve in us. Belden Lane writes that narrative is the most characteristic way of articulating any human experience.[9] We are always telling stories, making meaning of our lives in our stories. Stories can be written for ourselves (e.g., a diary or personal journal), but most narratives are intended for sharing with another something of ourselves and something of what holds meaning for us. Circumstances and contexts shape and form our stories. Once told, our story can also be shaped by the engagement of others with whom we share. Others may see something we missed. We may also, in time, see the story's significance differently. We come to know one another (and ourselves) through our stories. And just as memories include the dangerous and the delightful, so too do narratives.

When we tell our stories in light of the Christian story, new insights open up. When Christians hear and reflect on the stories of Jesus, the stories can help us see our own story differently. Our moral imagination becomes engaged. The same is true when we as a community of believers share our faith stories.[10] If memory is about identity, then narratives are the meaning makers of our identity. Robert Schreiter writes:

> [S]tories are powerful means for shaping our identities. They weave together in a narrative the events that have special significance for us . . .

Our identities are based strongly on the stories we tell about ourselves, our families, our communities, our countries. In these collections, stories about origins hold a special place. They embody the fundamental values that we see unfolding in the rest of our history . . . Significant too about the best of our stories is that they can be recast as our contexts change and as we gain new insights into ourselves and our communities. That does not mean that they are total fabrications or are completely subject to our whims. It means, rather, that they are not just accounts of the past, but are living parts of us now. The retelling of the stories is not so much about changing them as it is about gaining new perspective. Often that new perspective helps us understand our current situation better.[11]

If, then, hope is kept alive by memories and passed on in narratives, narratives are our stories of hope, even in the midst of suffering. Metz reminds us that "Christianity began as a community which remembered and told stories in the footsteps of Jesus, whose first gaze was not directed to the sin of others but to the suffering of others. This sensitivity to the suffering of others, this heeding of the suffering of others—including the suffering of enemies—in Jesus' own action lies at the center of that 'new way of living' which is associated with him. It is the most convincing expression of that love which Jesus entrusted to us and asked of us when—completely in line with his Jewish heritage—he invoked the unity of the love of God and love of neighbor."[12] "Dangerous narratives" evoke hope, yet they do not avoid suffering and loss. Hope, as we discovered in our discussion of the virtues, acknowledges the reality of what is, yet does not see that as the end of the story, and so leaves room for "another way."

When stories are shared, they have the potential to transform both the narrator and the listener. This happens in the telling and listening as well as in the engagement that flows from the narration. However, before going into what this potential for transformation might look like, let us discuss for a moment what is necessary for the sharing of our narratives, especially difficult or challenging ones, in a faith community.

HOSPITALITY

A community and a hospitable space are essential for sharing our narratives. If as disciples we truly wish to respond to the suffering of others, especially of those outside the margins, we must be persons and communities of hospitality. Although hospitality requires several things, only a few elements will be mentioned here.

First, hospitality demands that we be a community and a people *without borders*. Borders, ideological or concrete, are meant to keep some people in and some people out, or, at the least to keep track of "outsiders" coming in.[13] Borders presume that the other is a stranger rather than a neighbor, yet as disciples we are to treat the other as guest and neighbor rather than as stranger. People's experiences may differ greatly, and these experiences are to be seen as the gift each person and "stranger" brings to the community. It is a gift that must be honored as a sacred trust. Therefore, a sense of safety and trust is necessary for self-care and for care of the other to be held in faithful tension. In all, as disciples we are called to be "living embodiments of welcome."[14]

Narratives necessitate *presence* marked by a deep and *embodied listening* and *sharing*. When we invite a guest to share her story, we must be present in all possible ways to the person. In telling her story, the guest is offering us a part of her identity. In the sharing her identity intertwines with ours; she becomes a member of our community and we a part of her community. Thus, in the gathering and in the sharing, community is being transformed. It is significant to note that the *agency* of the guest is active in her *participation* in the community. As embodied persons we strive to open all of our senses as we hear and feel the narrative, a story that may include suffering and loss as well as survival and triumph over adversity.

We must also not be too quick to listen only for the "good news" of the story. We need to lament with the person as he relates his struggles. We must be aware that not all narrators have come down from the cross. The stories may open some listeners to seeing the crosses upon which too many people still hang today. The narrative may be calling us to stand with the other at the cross in mourning. The suffering may have no redemption at all, and to speak too quickly of redemption would be to deny the person's pain and even hinder his or her ability to move off the cross and through the pain to another moment beyond the pain. At this moment mercy simply calls us to enter into the chaos of the other's life with great care and respect.[15]

Hospitality requires a stance that honors the guest where he is. The community is asked to walk with the narrator wherever she is on her journey. For people who live on the margins, this accompaniment is prophetic and can be transformative. The narrator and the narrative are shaped by the experience of being heard. For listeners attentive to experiences on the margins and to the pain of their own lives, such accompaniment is the beginning of solidarity

A transformative spirit emerges in this kind of sharing. In the listening to and relating of the narrative, connections occur within the community. Even in grief, there is a possibility that narratives make all persons part of a community of hope. Sharing our stories liberates both individuals and communities. Stories remind us of our own lives and of our own "dangerous narratives" of suffering, hope, and resistance. Engaged listeners are caught up in spirit; the story becomes part of their own narrative and of their community's narrative as all are invited to share and engage. Even if the other is suffering, the narrative has the potential to become "good news;" the sharing signifies that the story has not ended but now continues with a living community of believers. Great freedom can emerge in voicing one's experiences of pain. Hilkert states this well when commenting on the blessing and importance of emerging women's voices: "The experience of women finding their voices, breaking the silence, and speaking with authority is part of the liberating good news that the gospel promises."[16]

Within a community of disciples, the faith narratives of scripture are woven into the listening and telling of our narratives, helping us to explore further layers of meaning. Lane reminds us that narratives have a "surplus of meaning" and are never exhausted in one telling.[17] We are people of the "Word," and our personal narratives interact with the "dangerous narratives" of Christian tradition, evoked in our liturgical life and in our biblical heritage. Narratives are part of an emerging tapestry that invokes the moral imagination and breaks open new possibilities. These narratives are truly "dangerous" for all because all belong in an inclusive circle that continues to widen. A circle of concern is embodied in a living community of hope. And hope, which is outside of us as well as within us, now has a hospitable space from which to speak, to envision, and to lead.

Hilkert reminds us that "the symbols and stories of our Christian hope 'capture the imagination' only when they are enfleshed in living communities of hope and resistance. Jesus did not proclaim the reign of God only in words; he enfleshed the good news he announced."[18] We are called, as disciples, to embody the good news and to name the incarnation we see in one another. This requires the sharing of stories of pain and suffering as well as of triumph and healing.

The sharing of narratives demands a response and engagement. The participation of all is engaged and demanded. Such engagement comes in many forms. When some share their narratives of suffering, enduring, and even of overcoming obstacles, the community laments with the one who suffers and rejoices with those who surmount obstacles.[19] The community also helps the one suffering endure when the loss or suffering cannot be removed; hope here is incarnated by the presence and support of those who commit to walking with us. What we have begun discussing is solidarity, to which we now turn.

SOLIDARITY

Eleanor Roosevelt is said to have once remarked, "My interest or sympathy or indignation is not aroused by an abstract cause but by the plight of a single person . . . Out of my response to an individual develops an awareness of a problem to the community, then to the country, and finally to the world. In each case my feeling of obligation to do something stemmed from one individual and then widened and became applied to a broader area."[20] Her response illustrates the powerful effect of knowing someone's story. In a very direct way we are moved beyond ourselves toward the other. What that way looks like encompasses many paths of solidarity. Memories articulated and shared through narratives have the power to evoke a response on behalf of the other. They help us pause for a moment to listen, to widen our circle of concern and make us readier to risk. They help ease us out of our personal and communal paralysis. The responses of solidarity are invitations to transformation and resurrection for all.

In defining solidarity, Roberto Goizueta writes: "in order to truly serve the neighbor, [that] love must be born out of an identification or solidarity with the neighbor in his or her joys, suffering, and struggles. The call to solidarity is a call to affirm in one's life the interdependence and unity of humankind before God; what happens to one happens to all."[21] Solidarity identifies us with one another, as we honor each "other" as embodied agents, even while connected by the bonds of our common humanity. Spohn writes that solidarity challenges any tendency to identify ourselves exclusively with any one community.[22] In creating a space of hospitality where there are no permanent borders, the sharing of narratives is actually an act of solidarity. As disciples, caring for the neighbor is a response to the love that has been given to us by God. Solidarity is here an effort to reflect humanly the mutuality and communion found in our teachings on the Trinity.[23]

Church documents and liberation theologies closely connect solidarity to people on the margins of society. Goizueta writes: "If solidarity implies an affirmation of human community, then it implies a special affirmation of those persons who have historically been excluded or ostracized from the human community: the hungry, the naked, the sick, the 'least ones' (see Mt. 25:31–46). Chapter 25 of Matthew's Gospel speaks of Jesus Christ's identification with the powerless; hence the Christian's identification with Jesus Christ is verified by his or her own identification with the powerless."[24] Because our community now includes the margins, an affirmation of persons requires that we go to the margins. We are to recreate communities without borders. "Margins," in whatever form, now threaten our unity and interdependence. In narratives we ask the question, "What are you going through?" and we listen to the response.[25] As we seek to relate to one another in solidarity, we, like Metz, transform the question "For what dare I hope?" to "For what dare I hope for you and, in the end, for me?"[26] The circle of concern is widened as we see our interrelatedness.

Solidarity on the "margins" teaches us several things. Solidarity reminds us of our mutual need for one another as a constitutive dimension of our humanity. Our humanity is connected with our fully embodied relational agency. In his encyclical *On Social Concern*, Pope John Paul II states: "Solidarity helps us to see the 'other'—whether a *person, people, or nation*—not just as some kind of instrument, with a work capacity or physical strength to be exploited at low cost and then discarded when no longer useful, but as our 'neighbor,' a 'helper' (cf. Gen. 2:18–20), to be made a sharer, on a par with ourselves, in the banquet of life to which we are all equally invited by God."[27] Reflective of our theological anthropology, Sobrino writes that the church has been "an instrument for giving voice to the cry of the poor majority, who by their very existence are trumpeting the proclamation that today one cannot be a human being *and* disregard the sufferings of millions of other human beings."[28] Our humanity is essentially connected to our interdependence, and so our hope is also connected to our solidarity.

This interdependence is at times surprising when we are "inside" the margins, for we may think that entering into solidarity with the poor and suffering puts us in a privileged "giving" stance and the other is, even in the most respectful fashion, in a stance of "receiving." Sobrino, however, writes powerfully that responding to the suffering of the poor is not only an ethical demand but that it is a "practice that is salvific for those who enter into solidarity with the poor. Those who do so often recover in their own life the deep meaning they thought they had lost; they recover their human dignity by becoming integrated into the pain and suffering of the poor. From the poor they receive, in a way they hardly expected, new eyes for seeing the ultimate truth of things and new energies for exploring unknown and dangerous paths. For them the poor are 'others,' and when they take on solidarity with them they undergo the experience of being sent to others only to find their own truth. At the very moment of giving they find themselves expressing gratitude for something new and better that they have been given."[29] All can find meaning and hope in the mutual interaction.

Solidarity reminds us that our hope and faith have a social character. Sobrino writes: "The root of solidarity is accordingly to be found in what generates human co-responsibility, makes co-responsibility an imperious ethical demand, and makes the exercises of co-responsibility something good, fulfilling, and salvific."[30]

Solidarity reveals to us the larger context and reality of injustice and evil, and, in turn, our co-responsibility. We gain valuable information by asking someone "What are you going through?" While the person may not necessarily have a prescription and procedure for what must be done, we learn essential data about the context in which something must be done.[31] Goizueta reminds us: "Solidarity with the powerless and an identification with their suffering reveal the many ways in which human beings continue to deny and undermine the unity of the human family, thereby denying the Creator."[32]

The perspective from which to look at suffering includes questions about the structural dimensions of the problem at hand. Patrick reminds us again that liberationist and feminist perspectives recognize the great extent to which *systemic* injustice causes suffering: "This means that the gift of 'food' and 'drink' should not be limited to the alleviation of immediate symptoms; we must also address the root causes of the unjust distribution of what is needed for our neighbors to flourish. Thus, from a feminist-liberationist perspective, there will be a priority of attention given to those whose lives are most harmed by racism, sexism, violence, and economic injustice."[33] On a systemic level, John Paul II calls for a move from an identification with the suffering to a practical response of correcting unjust structures.[34] Ada María Isasi-Díaz adds that in the midst of so much structural injustice the "goal is not the participation of the oppressed in present social structures but rather the replacement of those structures by ones in which full participation of the oppressed is possible."[35] This invites any number of ways to increase participation.

From our earlier discussions on situations of structural injustice related to HIV/AIDS, we know the significant damage that gender inequality, poverty, and structural injustice do to individuals, communities, nations, and continents. *That* we respond to the suffering in our world is a clarion call of discipleship. *That* solidarity calls the entire church community to respond in love and justice to our world today is clear. *How* we respond contains as many possibilities as we are willing to imagine and realize. The complexity of factors related to massive suffering invites and calls for a variety of ways to respond. *How exactly* you, I, and we are to respond emerges as we engage persons, needs, possibilities, and opportunities.

Dangerous memories interpreted through dangerous narratives of our tradition and of our lives lead us to solidarity as a stance and as an act. This in turn evokes the moral imagination and brings forth new possibilities. Our responses will be the result of the interaction we are entering into with our whole, embodied selves. And though we may take individual actions, we do not do this entirely by ourselves. We are a community, and we need the community to sustain us in the long haul of bringing about the Reign of God.

Earlier in this section on solidarity I said that "The responses of solidarity are invitations to transformation and resurrection for all." We explored this in terms of mutuality and co-responsibility for one another as we lament, hope, and respond as embodied, relational agents seeking to create borderless communities in a world of massive human suffering.

I end this section with a caution and a hope. The caution is that transformation or resurrection is not a guarantee when we encounter human suffering. Human suffering is not necessarily redemptive, and transformation is not a given, automatic result of solidarity with the one suffering. What the human body and spirit encounter in dire or tragic circumstances is often unfathomable, and there are times when reaching out does not happen soon enough.[36] We cannot forget the tragic dimensions of suffering because it is our dying, too. At the same time, there is always a transformative possibility when we reach out and engage one another. At times the spark of hope can live on very little.

The hope we have is a hope of the resurrection, and we have to embody the spirit of these narratives, share these narratives, and take on the challenges of these narratives on their multiplicity of levels. This is the hope of the resurrection. Resurrection here does not replicate the past but brings forth something new. Creative possibilities emerge from hope and resurrection. In terms of what can happen in the midst of solidarity rooted in dangerous memories and dangerous narratives, we again find insight from Schreiter. He describes resurrection as a "dynamic and transforming energy that does more than reconstitute things as they were before. It brings an utter transfiguration of beings."[37] As we mentioned earlier, Jesus' wounds remain after his resurrection, and he points them out to Thomas and to the other disciples when he appears to them. The suffering is not forgotten, but a transformation has occurred. Perhaps this is what happens when the community also allows itself to be transformed. All become living witnesses of the resurrection, an image not simply of "what Jesus would do" but an embodiment of "what Jesus is doing now."

Memory, narrative, and solidarity offer us a means of responding to people and to a world suffering with AIDS. Through these categories and practices, our frenetic activity, contextualized communities, and risk-averse society have a perspective from which to see, listen, pray, and act. These categories offer a positive response to our obstacles and pilot us on the road to discipleship.

QUESTIONS FOR REFLECTION AND DISCUSSION

1. What "dangerous memory" has affected your life? Is there a dangerous memory of scripture that you connect with your experience? What insights open up when you consider your dangererous memory in light of the Christian story?
2. What is a "dangerous memory" of scripture for you?
3. When have you heard a powerful narrative? What made the narrative so powerful?
4. Think of a time when you were in a gathering where people shared pain or vulnerability through their stories. How would you describe the listeners? What kind of environment do you think would be most helpful for welcoming a person with HIV/AIDS to share his or her story?
5. Has someone's story ever moved you to solidarity? If yes, how? If no, ask among your family and friends for any example they might have.
6. What might solidarity in an age of AIDS look like for you at this time?

CHAPTER 7

Bearing Witness:
Noerine Kaleeba and Paul Farmer

The test of our fundamental ethics, from anthropology to virtues to spirituality and morality, is how we respond to people and systems affected by the
HIV/AIDS pandemic. After considering elements of that discipleship which
flows from a response to our God and our neighbor and which is the proper
name for the unity between spirituality and morality, we considered strategies to keep the disciple open to the Gospel and to the world in the midst of
challenges to discipleship. We called these tools memory, narrative, and solidarity. Now we must ask ourselves whether these tools are adequate. Do
they sufficiently illuminate the world around us and serve as a way for the
disciple to respond to the suffering of people with AIDS around the world?

To begin to address this question I will examine two cases from the perspective of memory, narrative, and solidarity. The examples are of people
who bring a faith commitment to the situation of HIV/AIDS. The people
and groups are all responding to the HIV/AIDS pandemic. Each person is
Roman Catholic, and each person's ministry is ecumenical. In examining
each case, I will first relate the person's life as it intersects with the reality
of HIV/AIDS. I will then offer a brief analysis and assessment of each case in
terms of our discussions of theological anthropology, virtues, and discipleship. In doing so I will highlight the contributions each person makes and
what further responses each person calls forth from us as we consider fundamental ethics in our age of AIDS.

One final note of introduction: the Kaleeba and Farmer narratives are
invaluable conversation partners and are critical to constructing a fundamental ethics in an age of AIDS for a number of reasons. First, these are actual
cases of people today who are actively addressing the HIV/AIDS crisis in
various parts of the globe. They illuminate well the current situation in its
personal, interpersonal, and institutional dimensions. Second, these cases
offer an interpretive perspective from which to consider an embodied relational anthropology. Any attempt to construct a response to the HIV/AIDS

83

crisis benefits from efforts to interpret the lives of those who are actively engaged in HIV prevention and treatment efforts. Third, these cases are diverse enough to allow us to assess efforts toward transcultural and contextual sensitivity. Fourth, these cases dialogically engage the theological anthropology and discipleship proposed.

NOERINE KALEEBA: HOPE IN A TIME OF AIDS

Our first case begins in Uganda with the story of Noerine Kaleeba.[1] Noerine and Chris Kaleeba were married in 1975 and had four children. Noerine was a physiotherapist in Mulago hospital, a major hospital in Kampala. Chris worked in Adult Education and eventually received a scholarship to do graduate work in Britain at Hull University. He left in July 1985. On June 6, 1986, Noerine received news that Chris was seriously ill and in a Hull hospital. During a phone conversation with a doctor treating Chris, she was told that Chris tested positive for HIV and that he had AIDS.

Noerine was shocked by the news that Chris had AIDS, and before leaving for England to be with Chris, she shared the news with family, friends, neighbors, and colleagues at work. She was to later pay a price for sharing this news. At the London hospital where Chris was being treated, she found a loving and caring medical community and a Catholic chaplain.[2] They offered her the support, comfort, and counseling she needed to accept Chris's diagnosis and prognosis. While staying in London, Noerine took time to learn as much as she could about AIDS.

In September 1986, Noerine returned to Uganda because her daughters also needed her. Upon her return, she found that many people began to shun her and her daughters. There was more fear than education around AIDS, and people feared that HIV is infectious in the same way that measles is. Later in the year Chris's health improved enough for him to return to Uganda. However, when his health deteriorated again he was taken to Mulago hospital, and there again Noerine encountered stigma. Noerine reflected on this experience in an address to the World Health Assembly in May 2001: "I could not understand the basis of this stigma and it made me very angry. I felt very betrayed by the negative attitudes of health care workers who are the very persons supposed to restore people to health. It took me time to understand that the emergency of this new disease—for which there was very scanty information—was creating panic. This panic, combined with the fact that the disease was associated with the two taboo subjects of sex and death, was the source of the stigma."[3] The family decided to take Chris out of the hospital and bring him home, where he would be in the loving company of his family. It was there that some family and friends came and offered support.

A new source of support that emerged for Noerine and Chris came from a small group of people, twelve of whom were also affected by AIDS.[4] In January of 1987 Chris died of AIDS-related meningitis. This was a devastating time for Noerine on a number of levels. Kevin Kelly, who met Noerine in Kampala, explains, "Noerine was totally devastated by his death, by the terrible pain in which he died and by the way she and her daughters had been treated. To make matters worse, although Chris had made a will, it was not sufficiently specific to override local custom. Consequently, in accordance with the patriarchal traditions of her culture, the house in which Noerine and her daughters were living and the bit of land that went with it did not go to her and her children but to her husband's brother."[5] These experiences made clear to Noerine that much was wrong with the way Uganda was dealing with AIDS. Medical care was awful, and ignorance about AIDS was creating a great deal of fear among people across all educational, economic, gender, and religious lines. The subordination of women on several levels added further burdens when they or their family members were affected by AIDS.[6]

In November of 1987, Kaleeba and the sixteen members of her support group came together and decided to try to address some of these issues. Thus began TASO (The AIDS Support Organization). The group specifically put AIDS in the name of the organization as an effort to break the silence and stigma associated with AIDS.[7] John Mary Waliggo writes that Kaleeba names four factors crucial to the founding of TASO: "her strong belief in God's love and power; the fact that she was still healthy and therefore had a mission to realize; the gift of her four daughters whom she wanted to grow up as caring people; and the gift of friends with whom she wanted to be committed to a special mission."[8] Her faith, family, friends, and sense of mission would continue to be galvanizing factors in her life.

TASO was Uganda's first AIDS support group. Its activities grew from a small gathering of persons offering one another support to an organization that took on the multidimensional challenges of AIDS in a positive and holistic manner. TASO's activities generally were "sensitization and advocacy; training counselors at various levels of society; giving counseling to people infected and affected by AIDS; providing medical services; and, carrying out social welfare services."[9] An important slogan for TASO is "living positively with AIDS." This essential attitude emphasizes that there is hope and a way to live with the virus. In an address, "Stigma and AIDS," Kaleeba highlighted that promoting positive living is necessary for countering fatalistic tendencies prevalent in areas so devastated by AIDS. As an example, she took out a picture of primary school children leaving school and related: "In the picture of 45, only five are left. This level of impact, if we are not careful, can lead to fatalistic tendencies. 'What is your message? I don't even believe your messages. Look at how many have died, are dying.' We need to focus on where we can make a difference. We don't see new infections going down, but on the number of deaths occurring."[10]

TASO offers a hopeful interruption in a milieu in which it was believed that an HIV/AIDS diagnosis was simply a death sentence.[11] Counseling infected and affected persons about how to live positively with HIV/AIDS continues to be the heart of its mission.[12] Persons with HIV are encouraged to live responsibly. They are to make sure that they not spread their infection to another, maintain their health as much as possible, and stay connected with society.[13] At the same time, "living positively with AIDS" is each person's call, and therefore offering acceptance of persons with HIV/AIDS and offering support so that they can live well and fulfill their family responsibilities are important.

The approach of compassionate care within a supportive environment that seeks to eliminate discrimination and stigma through education and advocacy was a milestone in the treatment of HIV/AIDS in Uganda. Supported by the Ugandan government and subsequently adopted in other regions of the country, TASO's model educated the government, educational, social service, and health care organizations as well as religious bodies.[14] An ecumenical effort, TASO invites all people and all faiths. Kaleeba relates that TASO began as a group gathering to offer support, "praying and crying together. Although many of our founding members were practicing Christians, we made it a point to focus on practical issues in people's lives—regardless of whether they had faith or not."[15] That some family and friends objected to Chris because of his Protestant religion also made Kaleeba more sensitive to and accepting of people of all faiths.

Kaleeba served as director of TASO until 1995. TASO training now includes regions beyond Uganda, including, among others, Kenya, Tanzania, Rwanda, Malawi, Zambia, Zimbabwe, and Botswana. In 1996 she was offered a job with UNAIDS in Geneva to work as the Program Development Advisor in the Division for Africa. Of this opportunity, Kaleeba writes: "After leading the Ugandan AIDS movement for 10 years, I felt a strong need to influence global policy with experiences from my community."[16] She continues her work now with community development programs in areas such as northern Thailand, Cambodia, India, and Brazil.[17]

Analysis

Noerine Kaleeba's story offers hope in our age of AIDS. Her life speaks of an integration of memory, narrative, and solidarity in a way that includes all people as agents leading lives of meaning and hope. Kaleeba does not turn her back on the past or current suffering of persons with AIDS. Instead, she faces the situation with a love and compassion that seek to address the suffering in any way possible. Kaleeba's example calls others to steep themselves in the virtues of fidelity, justice, self-care, and prudence, and all this within the virtue of hope. She advocates for a range of involvement that includes each person and each system, for all are connected. She addresses the personal as well as the systemic issues related to and contributing to HIV/AIDS, touching on all the areas we have also discussed, including gender inequality and structural injustice. She has found ways to support people to address behavior that contributes to AIDS. She has worked and succeeded in influencing governments and international organizations to support and provide prevention and treatment efforts.

Kaleeba's memories are truly dangerous. She experienced the compassion and support of health care workers and a Catholic chaplain in London when she and Chris struggled to confront AIDS. She also experienced stigma and isolation in Uganda from the very persons from whom she expected comfort and understanding. Through all this she found comfort and strength in her faith. Her memories included time in prayer with people who came to offer one another support. She found herself on the margins of society in a way she never imagined, and she knew the challenges of AIDS from very personal experiences. She also knew something of what was helpful to her in the midst of the challenges. Noerine's memories continue to give life to her husband Chris and to the many she meets who struggle with AIDS.

The memories became narratives as they were shared. Kaleeba's life was shared with others who gathered with her, and all shared their circumstances as they tried to support one another. These narratives were told in the context of prayer, and both lamentation and sass emerged. In the gatherings there was a borderless hospitality. Especially welcome were the vulnerable, ostracized, sick, and needy. A new community was formed, one which countered the fear and discrimination around AIDS in the community and the nation at large.

It was in the gathering to share with one another that a hopeful imagination led to the founding of TASO. Narratives continue to be powerful tools for TASO and for many prevention and advocacy efforts. In many of Kaleeba's writings and speeches she shares her story and stories of people infected or affected by AIDS. She exhorts people and groups to listen to these narratives and those of others struggling with AIDS, for it is here that insights about prevention, care, and support are also to be found. In a speech to the World Health Assembly in 2001, she appealed to the group: "First, find the space and time to listen to people affected by HIV. Because if you do, you will find out that they are your key allies in the HIV/AIDS response. Their concerns are also your concerns—namely their health and human rights and the future of their children."[18] The narratives are of hope as well as of great challenge. The narratives are also a way of keeping alive those who have died, sustaining their memory in gatherings to support one another and to promote a future without AIDS.

TASO is an excellent example of how memories and narratives can galvanize solidarity.[19] The solidarity promoted by TASO is with all people, and especially with those infected and affected by HIV/AIDS. A vision and mission emerged for Kaleeba and for others who gathered and shared their stories. TASO was the first such support group in Uganda, and it emerged from experiences and evident needs. From a small group supporting one another in their personal struggles with AIDS-related problems came organizing efforts such as counseling for individuals and families, helping people with basic health care needs, and educating people about HIV/AIDS and prevention.

Solidarity grew as communities and the government saw the necessity and benefit of TASO's programs. This changed both individual lives and the life of a nation and its government. The solidarity Kaleeba and TASO and UNAIDS promote includes all dimensions of living. These efforts promote hope through responsibility for and responsiveness to the challenges and needs of a world with AIDS. Such solidarity affirms that each person and group has something to offer in a situation that requires multidimensional efforts ranging from the spiritual and religious to the socioeconomic, political, and cultural. Discipleship includes all of these dimensions.

Noerine Kaleeba offers a solid example of grass-roots efforts to react to the personal circumstances of HIV/AIDS in a way that responds to the communal crisis of AIDS. Her efforts are rooted in a vision of the person as an embodied, relational agent, and she calls communities to this vision. She does not run from suffering, but recognizes it and seeks to address its causes on personal and structural levels today. Her efforts model discipleship, flowing from a vision of what humans are and need and of how they can best flourish together.

Kaleeba challenges all people to involve themselves in the crisis of AIDS and uses her memories, her narratives, and the narratives of others to invite further efforts of solidarity. A strength of TASO is that it includes all religions and faiths. Waliggo underscores the importance of this as he writes that TASO is an exemplar of an "ecumenical, interfaith movement and organization. It helps to bring out the common denominators of all believers of God. The issues of human dignity, human equality, human rights; preferential care for the vulnerable, disadvantaged, marginalized, those in special need; issues of the compassion of God, God's loving care and forgiveness; the need for human solidarity and concern; the challenge against self-righteousness and judging others rashly all come to the fore in TASO."[20] Kaleeba models a discipleship which seeks to permeate boundaries between religions, cultures, economics, and geography and includes all in realizing the great human dignity of each and all. She is an embodiment of hope in our age of AIDS.

PAUL FARMER: "WE'RE ALL HUMAN BEINGS"

At the age of twenty-three, after graduating from college and before going to medical school, Paul Farmer spent some time volunteering as a doctor's assistant in a hospital in Leogane, in Haiti.[21] One day he had a long conversation with an American doctor who was returning to the United States after working for a year among the people of Haiti. When Farmer asked him if he was finding it hard to leave, the doctor replied that he could hardly wait to leave, for conditions in Haiti were brutal. Farmer, observing that the doctor seemed to love the people, pressed further. "But aren't you worried about not being able to forget all this? There's so much disease here." The doctor's response was "No. I'm an American and I'm going home."[22] Farmer thought about that response the rest of the day, wondering "What does that mean, 'I'm an American?' How do people classify themselves?"[23]

That night a young pregnant woman with a severe case of malaria came to the hospital. She went into a coma and needed a blood transfusion. However, there was no blood at the hospital and the doctor told the woman's sister to go to Port-au-Prince to get some blood. The sister had no money for blood and so Farmer rounded up fifteen dollars and gave it to her. The woman left and then returned because she did not have enough money to go to Port-au-Prince. In the midst of this, the patient went into respiratory distress and died. She was the mother of five children. The sister said, "This is terrible. You can't even get a blood transfusion if you're poor . . . We're all human beings." Over and over again she kept saying, "We're all human beings."[24] Farmer cried as he shared this story from over twenty years ago. That refrain remains with him today.

In 1984, following this experience, Farmer enrolled in medical school at Harvard. He graduated with a medical degree and a Ph.D. in anthropology in 1990. Even during graduate school he was often in Haiti. In the Central Plateau and the village of Cange he helped to slowly create a medical complex that would be called Zanmi Lasante, Creole for "Partners in Health."[25] And in 1987 he and a number of American friends founded Partners in Health (PIH), the sponsoring organization of Zanmi Lasante.[26] Zanmi Lasante and PIH collaborated on a number of projects addressing areas ranging from AIDS, tuberculosis, and maternal mortality to malnutrition and illiteracy.[27] Though Zanmi Lasante is the largest sister organization, PIH collaborates with a number of other projects, including Socios En Salud, a primary health care program in Carabayllo, Peru; Haitian Teens Confront AIDS, a Boston-area AIDS prevention program for young Haitians; Soldiers of Health, a community-based project for health and well-being for people with poor access to quality health care; Apoyo A Mujeres and Guatemalan Refugee Project in Chiapas, Mexico, for refugees and indigenous Chiapanecos for women's health care and to develop community health training and support services.[28]

The logo for PIH consists of four intersecting hands and the slogan "Making a Preferential Option for the Poor in Health Care." The aim of PIH is explained well in the PIH brochure: "People living in poverty seldom need outside help to identify the nature of their problems. What they lack are the material resources to address them. For these reasons, we regard our task as primarily a pragmatic one. Through 'pragmatic solidarity' with our partners, our goals are to: 1. improve the health of the poor and their communities; 2. foster active community involvement in the planning and implementation of efforts to maintain health and overcome illness; and 3. expose the structures that create vast disparities in access to medical care and, ultimately, join hands with those who seek to change them."[29] The invitation of PIH is to all.

Analysis

For our purposes it is important to note the theological underpinning particularly evident in the slogan and goals of PIH. A "preferential option for the poor" is a clarion cry both of liberation theology and of the Catholic social tradition, and Paul Farmer has taken this call seriously, bringing it to his practice of medicine and to the wider medical community as well as to the world and Church community. Farmer is well versed in liberation theology and acknowledges its influence on the plans and efforts of Partners in Health.[30] In an article written for *America* and based on a lecture at Creighton University, Farmer explores what a health intervention inspired by liberation theology might look like.[31] Engaging insights from Leonardo Boff, Jon Sobrino, Gustavo Gutiérrez, Paulo Freire, and documents from the Medellín (1968) and Puebla (1978) conferences, he utilizes liberation theology's three-part methodology of "observe, judge and act," and he sees social justice as the necessary response. His own memories and the narratives of those he serves are engaged with an analysis of the sociopolitical, economic, cultural, religious, and medical situation of the people. The observations, research, and analysis lead to the conclusion that something is very wrong when the poor are at "heightened risk of dying prematurely, whether from increased exposure to pathogens (including pathogenic situations) or from decreased access to services or, as is most often the case, from both of these 'risk factors.'"[32]

Liberation theology emphasizes analyzing the root causes of health problems and bringing forth the experiences and insights from the poor into all the ways that one sees, judges, and acts. Farmer sees the root causes of health problems as being found in structural injustices that permit and even promote an inequity that allows the poor to die of illnesses for which there are effective treatments.[33] He cites in agreement Boff's declaration that "'the church's option is a preferential option *for the poor, against their poverty.*' The poor, Boff adds, 'are those who suffer injustice. Their poverty is produced by mechanisms of impoverishment and exploitation. Their poverty is therefore an evil and an injustice.'"[34] The response to structural injustices must be social justice, and one means of achieving this is pragmatic solidarity.

To choose an option for the poor is to work for social justice, and doing so means not only taking care of immediate needs but also working together to change the systems that are oppressive and that keep people poor. Working together puts a particular obligation on people of privilege and wealth of any sort, whether these are due to their education or influence or material resources. Farmer makes this clear when he states that a preferential option for the poor means that our analysis must be historically deep. This requires our memory to have historical roots. In the situation of Haiti, the poorest country in our hemisphere, the United States needs to remember that "modern-day Haitians are the descendants of a people kidnapped from Africa in order to provide us with sugar, coffee and cotton."[35] He also writes that our analysis must be geographically broad, for to appreciate a world that is increasingly interconnected is to understand that in health care or otherwise, "what happens to poor people is never divorced from the actions of the powerful. Certainly, people who define themselves as poor may control to some extent their own destinies. But control of lives is related to the control of land, systems of production and the formal political and legal structures in which lives are enmeshed. There has come, with time, an increasing concentration of wealth and control in the hands of the few."[36] He challenges all power structures on this topic, but he especially challenges the privileged everywhere, including those in the United States.

Social justice is Paul Farmer's prevailing message, and he brings this to the AIDS crisis as well. Presenting at the XIII International AIDS conference in Durban, South Africa, he noted the Joint United Nations Programme on HIV/AIDS, 2000, which reported an "increasing concentration of HIV among the poor and marginalized, most of them in the so-called developing countries" and which predicted that by the end of the decade over 95% of all AIDS deaths will occur in "resource-poor settings."[37] He argued that prevention and treatment strategies must be linked, and that both need a social justice component. While supporting education as an important prevention strategy, Farmer challenges its efficacy in a compromised environment:

Show us the data to suggest that, in settings where *social conditions* determine risk for HIV infection, cognitive exercises can fundamentally alter risk. We know that risk of acquiring HIV does not depend on knowledge of how the virus is transmitted, but rather on the freedom to make decisions. Poverty is the great limiting factor of freedom. Indeed, gender inequality and poverty are far more important contributors to HIV risk than is ignorance of modes of transmission or "cultural beliefs" about HIV. We can already show that many who acquire HIV infection do so *in spite of* knowing enough information to protect themselves, if indeed cognitive concerns were ever central to preventing HIV among the poor. Until we have effective, female-controlled prevention, whether a microbicide or another, and an effective vaccine, nothing we do should suggest that education can substitute for, or remove the necessity of, effective therapy for AIDS.[38]

Farmer challenges any who argue that HIV/AIDS treatment among the poor and in developing countries is "not sustainable" and notes the profits pharmaceutical companies are making while the poor are dying because they cannot afford treatment which can extend their lives and give their children more time to have a parent.[39] Farmer asserts again and again that the "struggle for social and economic rights for the poor must become central to every aspect of AIDS research and treatment."[40]

Farmer also brings this challenge to the Catholic tradition. He challenges local HIV prevention efforts to be connected to large-scale efforts. From over a decade of work in Haiti, Farmer makes the following observation and claim: "*If poverty and gender inequality conspire to increase HIV risks for poor women, then the promotion of social and economic rights must be central to HIV/AIDS prevention.* The press for fulfillment of these rights falls squarely within the magisterium of the church, which has to date failed to incorporate social-justice perspectives into its HIV/AIDS-prevention activities—such as they are."[41] Farmer challenges the Church to speak publicly of the connection between social inequality and HIV transmission and to actively work to remedy this situation. This of course requires the Church to confront gender and social inequality within its own community and practices. Farmer sees hope in the base communities of the Church for movements to confront inequalities in all areas of society.

While encouraging the Church to act to meet the needs of this time of AIDS, Farmer also demands that "*faith-based responses must be technically correct and based on sound analyses* . . . As far as AIDS goes, this often means questioning the 'immodest claims of causality' currently advanced to explain the failure of HIV/AIDS prevention among the poor. The default explanations have been the usual ones: the 'noncompliance' of the poor, their cultural particularities, their cognitive deficits. Each of these essentialist explanatory gambits locates the problem squarely within the poor: the problem lies with the poor, so HIV/AIDS-prevention efforts should change them rather than their circumstances."[42] Farmer challenges such an exaggeration of agency, again commenting on the social and economic situations of the poor and marginalized which remove any freedom of agency. These are important points for the Roman Catholic Church to note, particularly because the Church is a large nongovernment organization (NGO) in Africa.

The value of each person is crucial for Farmer, and his option for the poor is rooted in memories and experiences of the poor and marginalized being at risk. He is a North American and a U.S. citizen who actively asks how it is that the life and health of someone with wealth and resources is valued more than those of someone with less. That people anywhere are dying of treatable diseases is completely unacceptable.[43] He values an embodied relational agency, but sees that in the present economic and social circumstances, this is not a reality for the poor. For him, changing the socioeconomic situation of the poor would allow the possibility of embodied relational agency to become a reality.

Farmer's rhetoric also presumes that those with privilege and access have an embodied relational agency, but that it is sorely underutilized and impoverished. He encourages those of us who have privilege and access to respond to the AIDS crisis with a sense of relationality to those beyond even our experiences. The narratives he offers in almost every presentation and paper are a way to bridge the gap of understanding. He calls for a fully embodied response, and this includes our material resources, lobbying and voting resources, and our presence. Farmer challenges all, including the group he called "W.L.s"—white liberals—to realize that fixing the problems of the world will require a cost and a sacrifice to themselves.[44] Farmer knows he can have a life of privilege and like it, but he says he is not willing to "erase this world of suffering . . . People don't get up in the morning and say, 'I'm going to erase this world of suffering.' They're just cosseted. They don't have to see the suffering. We live in a country so rich that you can hide away anything in it. What does it mean to be human, as opposed to being American?"[45] He probes further, "My big struggle is how people can not care, erase, not remember."[46]

Farmer deals with this struggle by example. In addition to spending considerable time in Haiti in the clinical setting and serving as founding director of Partners in Health, Farmer is associate professor in two departments at the Harvard Medical School, senior staff member in Infectious Disease at Brigham and Women's Hospital in Boston, and chief consultant on tuberculosis in Russian prisons for the World Bank. He writes and presents nationally and internationally, bringing his message to the medical community as well as the church communities.

It was liberation theology's "powerful rebuke to the hiding away of poverty" that brought him back to Catholicism, yet this was after he was already immersed in Haiti.[47] His growing awareness of so much, including the impact that the power and privilege of one group had on the poor, "was a process, not an event. A slow awakening, as opposed to an epiphany."[48] The "pragmatic solidarity" he preaches flows from this process of memories in Haiti, narratives from the people he meets, and partnerships with all persons willing to work for the various goals that are constitutive of Partners in Health and Farmer's own mission. The memories are dangerous because he sees in them what must not be, and he is not willing to turn his back on the suffering. The narratives are dangerous because his work continues to be formed by them. He shares the people's dangerous narratives with those who are in "privileged positions" yet who do not face the suffering—and he challenges privileged persons and groups to see the suffering and respond. Paul Farmer's solidarity and that of Partners in Health are impressive because they utilize so many resources from the basic sciences, social sciences, theology, and many other areas to analyze and respond to foundational causes of health crises such as HIV/AIDS. Both see a connection between social issues and poor health, and both want the privileged to hear this. Desiring self-care for each person to be a reality, they especially want the privileged to be aware that self-care must be in proper relationship with the basic needs of many others in the world.

Farmer is conscious of his own conversion process. As he seeks to help form people's awareness and to galvanize a response to unjust living situations, his efforts to prevent persons and peoples from "being erased" continue. He challenges systems even as he responds to the daily demands of the sick. Aware of the Catholic Church's commitment to justice, he calls the institution and her people to embody what we say we believe. Farmer embodies justice; and his challenge continues to be how to get more people involved in social justice. He shares narratives and presents scientific facts, and by example he offers any number of creative options for involvement. Farmer's voice is in sync with the prophets of the Hebrew Scriptures, who continually prodded and at times forcefully challenged the community to remember the poor, the widowed, and the orphaned. Finally, Farmer embodies hope, for he brings it from his own experiences and he finds it in involvement with others.

We see in this chapter a spirituality and morality for this age of AIDS, and two examples of discipleship which incorporate memory, narrative, and solidarity. Both Noerine Kaleeba (and TASO) and Paul Farmer (and PIH) integrate in different ways the theological anthropology, virtues, and spirituality necessary to respond helpfully and hopefully in this age of AIDS.

QUESTIONS FOR REFLECTION AND DISCUSSION

1. What virtues does Noerine Kaleeba offer as a response to HIV/AIDS?
2. Find The AIDS Support Organization (TASO) on the internet at http://www.tasouganda.org. What elements of TASO would be helpful to your city or region today?
3. What insights into living one's faith and responding to people's needs does Paul Farmer offer you?
4. Explore the Partners in Health (PIH) website at http://www.pih.org/index.html.
5. What might a local response to HIV/AIDS look like at your school, institution, parish, or community center?
6. What services are available for people in your parish or diocese who are infected or affected by HIV/AIDS? Are there any unmet needs?

Conclusion: Now What?

In the beginning of this book I stated that I write about AIDS because God's people live with HIV/AIDS and because theology and ethics must be practiced in the midst of the people of God. It was perhaps only in the midst of writing that I truly realized the vastness of this topic! And I must admit to feeling almost overwhelmed every time I read the latest *UNAIDS Global Report*. How can the situation of so many people continue to deteriorate? And once the shock is over, it is the people affected and at risk of infection who continue to compel me. I keep near my desk a photo from my summer in Ghana. It is a picture of a number of the children I met in a remote village the summer my interest in AIDS was awakened. Their lives simultaneously hold so much potential—and so much risk—in our age of AIDS. They challenge me.

Once we realize that God's people have HIV/AIDS, we are all challenged with the Now what? What can I do? What can we do? And we must find some concrete, achievable answers to these questions—lest we freeze or walk away—if we are to sustain a response. Because our response must be multi-dimensional, short term, and long term, and utilize all available resources, all of our gifts must be brought to the table.

It would be very easy at the end of this book to simply place Noerine Kaleeba and Paul Farmer on pedestals as models of what is to be done, and then put this book and topic away. But pedestals are seductive. When we put people on pedestals we remove ourselves from the responsibility of stepping forward and doing something. We say that we can never become that person or do all that the other has done. But neither Farmer nor Kaleeba asks us to be like them or to put them on pedestals. We are only asked to do our part, to offer what we can. We cannot hold back, for just as Pope John Paul II often stated that "the poor cannot wait," so too God's people with HIV/AIDS cannot wait.

Our tradition of faith offers us stories of Jesus, and the moral imagination reminds us that we are called to follow Jesus in this our *kairos* time and place. God is in our historical *now*. Our relationship with God and others calls us more deeply and more fully into a world of joy as well as suffering. The spiritual and moral life become one as we do what would otherwise seem impossible—interrupt and stop the AIDS pandemic.

This is the conclusion to *When God's People Have HIV/AIDS*. You and I and we are the epilogue. We are the What Now.

I conclude by offering some suggestions about what can come next—and then invite both *your* engagement and further imaginative suggestions from *you*. When God's people have AIDS, all of God's people must respond.

1. *Begin with education.* More people need to know about God's people who have HIV/AIDS. People need good education about HIV/AIDS and the ethical issues inherent in the lives of people at risk for HIV/AIDS. Learn more and share this learning with others. Commit to knowing about the reality of AIDS in your state or country *and* in at least one other region of the world. Far too few colleges, universities, and parishes offer courses on this topic. Ask for a course in your school or parish and include some action components with the learning.

2. *Engage the global community.* It is crucial to engage with a global community of theologians, scholars, and activists. A richness of thought and possibility emerges when social location and experience are brought to theological discussions. Our conversations are further enriched when we engage not only through writing but also through listening to and discussing with persons from various parts of the world. We must especially listen to the people on the front lines of the HIV/AIDS epidemic. Seek out readings and conversation partners from a variety of places.

3. *Meet God's people who are living with HIV/AIDS.* Ask them to share their stories. Be willing also to share some of your own "dangerous memories." The elements of memory, narrative, and solidarity hold great promise for discernment within communities. How our communities engage memories and narratives (communal as well as personal) determines the direction our solidarity takes; the transformative potential is significant. An openness of the heart and the head is necessary for such transformation to solidarity. Pray for openness.

4. *Develop further the embodied relational agent in each culture and community.* The further I delve into theological anthropology, the more I realize that a consideration of an embodied relational agent in the context of historical suffering will continue to open layers of meaning for probing. Bringing this anthropology to life through the virtues and a consideration of discipleship is one way to mine its richness. However, the invitation is for further work in this anthropology. Each culture must enrich this anthropology for its particular community. What elements of the embodied relational person are at particular risk in a given community? In *your* community?

   The dimensions are diverse. I am particularly aware of the need for more development in the area of embodiment as it interconnects with spirituality. The anthropology must also be elaborated for each particular culture. I am keenly aware that more work must also be done toward a theology of marriage and of family in the midst of AIDS. The increasing devastation within families and among children must be addressed with all the theological, ecclesial, and pastoral resources available. Further interdisciplinary development in this area of relationality is crucial. Discuss with a variety of persons (gender, race, orientation, age, place of origin, etc.) the dimensions of the person that are at risk in your community and how you might positively address this risk. Name the ways that the person as embodied relational agent is affirmed and strengthened. Offer some individual and communal practices that affirm the person.

5. *Pray.* Take time to attend to God's word. As a Church, we must be grounded in contemplation. We must be women and men of prayer. As God's people we must be communities of faith, participating in personal, communal, and liturgical practices and allowing ourselves to be penetrated by the Spirit. We can only stay in the immediate and long-term struggle to help God's people with AIDS if we attend to our spiritual life. Take time to attend to God's word incarnated. In doing so, you open yourself to hearing the voice of God in the other in need.

6. *Participate in dialogue.* In our Church, dialogue on how to respond to God's people with HIV/AIDS must flow out of a contemplative stance, from which we respectfully listen to one another as members of the body of Christ. The first step is to listen. The current polarization among many groups within the Church (as well as in the United States and among various nations) creates missed opportunities to build relationships and forge commitments to eradicate HIV/AIDS. We must find ways to exchange ideas that are respectfully of the other, steeped in a common language of our Catholic tradition, in which we are able to critically engage one another's points for their strengths and seek to build upon the most each perspective offers in order to best respond to the needs of the suffering.[1]

We must engage in dialogue about our sexual lives. We need to discuss the pressures inherent in our lives today as bodily, sexual persons. We must discuss sexual ethics related to HIV/AIDS prevention. We must recognize the reality of so many women's broken bodies around the world. Wherever we see it, whether in our churches, our civil laws, or our private practices, we must recognize and resist the sins of sexism and classism, as well as any forms of discrimination based on race or sexual orientation. There must be no taboo topic, for from these honest discussions emerge our challenge and opportunity for responding to the reality of people's lives. We must call one another to our potential as God's creation and beloved and offer support on the journey.

Find someone whose perspective on an issue important to you may differ from yours. Begin a conversation with the intention of truly hearing that person's perspective in its best positive light. Invite the other to do the same.

7. *Find ways to act.* The Church must act. Our ecclesial communities must offer a social ethics "interruption" of AIDS prevention and treatment

conversations. Gender inequality and poverty are foundational contributing factors to the spread of HIV/AIDS. As citizens of the world and as men and women of faith, we dare not overlook or underestimate these factors that desperately need our engagement.

There is both blessing and responsibility in membership within a universal Church. There are dimensions of HIV/AIDS that the Church community can respond to simply because we are a global community called to serve the people of God. The concerns of God's people around the globe must be our concerns because these are also our communities. The global dimensions of AIDS demand continued ethical engagement with global arenas such as the pharmaceutical industry. In order to provide care and treatment for persons affected by HIV/AIDS, there is a need for greater collaboration with experts in areas such as economics, business, and medicine. This collaboration may also serve as a bridge by which our local Church communities can positively affect the many needs that AIDS devastation presents. Accept the blessing and responsibility that are yours as a member of the Church.

Choose and commit to one area of concern and get involved on a local and global level. Find a community or organization that is addressing this area and get involved.

8. *Imagine a world without AIDS.* AIDS need not exist. See an alternative reality to work toward. Act with others to eradicate HIV/AIDS. Share success stories, no matter how small. Good news generates further efforts and offers hope. Hope expands the horizons of the possible so that what is not may someday be—a world without AIDS.[2]

In closing, just as Metz could not practice theology with his back to the Holocaust, our generation cannot be a Church with our back to the faces of people with HIV/AIDS. Our generation cannot claim, "We did not know!" The vocation of the disciple is to read the "signs of the times" and to utilize resources to offer a positive response. Disciples cannot, if ever we could, labor in an ivory tower—for we have seen too many towers, fiscal and ecclesial, fall these past few years. Our efforts must be at the service of the wider community and our Church communities. This is the call and demand of discipleship.

QUESTIONS FOR REFLECTION AND DISCUSSION

1. What, now, will you do?
2. With whom?

Notes

Introduction

1. Unless otherwise indicated, in this introduction the names of people infected with HIV/AIDS have been changed to preserve confidentiality.

2. A group of women religious had started an educational and vocational school for poor "at risk" young girls so that they would receive an education (still deemed "unnecessary" for girls by some parents who would rather have the girls help in the fields) and gain the skills and self-confidence necessary to find work, which would offer economic stability.

3. While in El Salvador in December 2000, I heard married and unmarried women offer the same reasons of "culture, pleasure, and economics" for why their male partners did not use condoms. These are relatively common experiences, as can be seen in the literature. See, for example, Johanna McGreary, "Death Stalks a Continent," *Time*, 12 February 2001, 42; Laurenti Magesa, "Recognizing the Reality of African Religion in Tanzania," in *Catholic Ethicists on HIV/AIDS Prevention*, ed. James F. Keenan, assisted by Jon D. Fuller, Lisa Sowle Cahill, and Kevin Kelly (New York: Continuum, 2000), 76–84.

4. Joint United Nations Programme on HIV/AIDS (UNAIDS), Peter Piot, preface to *Report on the Global HIV/AIDS Epidemic, 2002*, 6; available at http://www.unaids.org/barcelona/presskit/barcelona%20report/preface.html; Internet; accessed 10 October 2002.

5. Ibid., 1.

6. Vatican Council II, *Gaudium et Spes*, in *Catholic Social Thought: The Documentary Heritage*, ed. David J. O'Brien and Thomas A. Shannon (Maryknoll, NY: Orbis, 1992), no. 4.

7. UNAIDS/WHO, *AIDS Epidemic Update: December 2004*, 2; available at http://www.unaids.org/wad2004/EPI_1204_pdf_en/EpiUpdate04_en.pdf; Internet; accessed 27 November 2004. Also, note that the ranges around the estimates "define the boundaries within which the actual numbers lie, based on the best available information."

1. Constructing a Fundamental Ethics

1. The indicators covered in this section are written to offer the reader a sense of what is at stake in the HIV/AIDS pandemic. The information that follows offers glimpses of the reality of HIV/AIDS, which we take with us as we explore a fundamental ethic in this age of AIDS.

2. National Institute of Allergy and Infectious Diseases (NIAID), *HIV Infection and AIDS*, March 1999, 1; available at http://www.aegis.com/topics/basics/whataidsis.html; Internet; accessed 2 December 1999.

3. Ibid.

4. Ibid. Recent reports indicate that HIV is spreading in rural parts of China because the poor are illegally selling their blood to "blood heads," who tend to use unsterile methods. See Elisabeth Rosenthal, "AIDS Scourge in Rural China Leaves Village of Orphans," *New York Times*, 25 October 2002.

5. Ibid. A challenge here is that many infants born to HIV/AIDS-infected mothers will die if they do not at least have the nutrition from breast milk. Without alternative nutrition, breast-feeding remains the only option.

6. UNAIDS/WHO, *2004 AIDS Epidemic Update: December 2004*,6; available at http://www.unaids.org/wad2004/EPI_1204_pdf_en/EpiUpdate04_en.pdf; Internet; accessed 27 November 2004.

7. Ibid., 3. The listing is from lowest numbers to highest numbers, with 2002 figures as the ordering base. A cautionary note regarding estimates is necessary here. Each listing of UNAIDS/WHO estimates is based on the most recent available data and the best available methods for deriving estimates. The estimates are provisional and the numbers are regularly reviewed and updated. Because of this, one cannot directly compare estimates from previous years with most recent years or even future years (see UNAIDS/WHO, "Explanatory Note about UNAIDS/WHO Estimates," in *AIDS Epidemic Update: December 2004*). With that proviso in mind, it is still helpful to see the estimates.

8. For the most up-to-date estimates, see the UNAIDS website at http://www.unaids.org. Reports and updates on the epidemic are published twice a year. Information for specific counties and regions is available. Information specific to the United States can also be found at the Center for Disease Control website at http://www.cdc.gov.

9. UNAIDS/WHO, *2004 AIDS Epidemic Update: December 2004*, 69, 70. However, the majority of persons in the United States living with HIV are still men who have sex with men.

10. Centers for Disease Control, *HIV/AIDS Surveillance Report* 15 (2004); CDC, "HIV/AIDS in America Today," presented by Dr. Harold Jaffe at the National HIV Prevention Conference, 2003. Cited in Henry J. Kaiser Family Foundation, "The HIV/AIDS Epidemic in the United States," HIV/AIDS Policy Fact Sheet, December 2004; available at http://www.kff.org; Internet; accessed 12 December 2004.

11. It is especially important to note reported infections among young people. Because they are more likely to have been recently exposed to HIV, this can indicate overall trends in incidence. UNAIDS/WHO, *AIDS Epidemic Update: December 2002*, 4–5, 27.

12. UNAIDS/WHO, *2004 AIDS Epidemic Update: December 2004*, 69.

13. Ibid. Centers for Disease Control and Prevention. *HIV/AIDS Among African-Americans*, 2003; available at http://www.cdc.gov/hiv/pubs/facts/afam.htm; Internet; accessed 27 December 2004. In addition, the December 2004 report states, "In 2003, African Americans accounted for at least 25% of all AIDS cases, compared with 20% in 2001. That proportion could be higher, since the estimate was based on data collected in just 20 states."

14. Center for Disease Control and Prevention, *HIV/AIDS Surveillance Report* 15 (2004); U.S. Census Bureau, *Annual Estimates of the Population by Sex, Race and*

Hispanic or Latino Origin for the United States: April 1, 2000 to July 1, 2003 (Washington, DC). Population estimates do not include U.S. dependencies, possessions, or associated nations. May not total 100% because of rounding; persons who reported more than one race were included in multiple categories.

15. CDC, *HIV/AIDS Surveillance Report* 15 (2004). Estimates do not include cases from the U.S. dependencies, possessions, or associated nations or cases of unknown residence. Cited in Henry J. Kaiser Family Foundation, "The HIV/AIDS epidemic in the United States," HIV/AIDS Policy Fact Sheet, December 2004, available at http://www.kff.org; Internet; accessed 12 December 2004.

16. UNAIDS/WHO, *AIDS Epidemic Update: December 2004*, 70.

17. UNAIDS/WHO, *AIDS Epidemic Update: December 2002*, 27.

18 UNAIDS/WHO, *2004 AIDS Epidemic Update: December 2004*, 69–70.

19. Ibid., 70.

20. Ibid. See also Centers for Disease Control and Prevention, "HIV/AIDS among African-Americans," Fact Sheet (Washington, DC: U.S. Centers for Disease Control and Prevention), available at http://www.cdc.gov/hiv/pubs/facts/afam.htm; Internet; accessed 16 September 2004; U.S. Census Bureau, *Poverty Status of the Population in 1999 by Age, Sex, and Race and Hispanic Origin* (Washington, DC: U.S. Census Bureau, 2000); T. Diaz et al., "Socioeconomic Differences among People with AIDS: Results from a Multistate Surveillance Project," *American Journal of Preventive Medicine* 10, no. 4 (1994): 217–22.

21. UNAIDS/WHO, *AIDS Epidemic Update: December 2004*, 71.

22. Ibid., 19.

23. Ibid.

24. UNAIDS, *Report on the Global HIV/AIDS Epidemic, July 2004*.

25. Ibid.

26. UNAIDS/WHO, *AIDS Epidemic Update: December 2004*, 25.

27. UNAIDS, *Report on the Global HIV/AIDS Epidemic, July 2004*.

28. UNAIDS/WHO, *AIDS Epidemic Update: December 2004*, 25.

29. Ibid., 26.

30. UNAIDS, "Report on the Global HIV/AIDS Epidemic—AIDS in a new millennium, 2000," online report, 5–6; available at www.unaids.org/epidemic_update/report/Epi_report_chap_millenium.htm.

31. UNAIDS/WHO, *AIDS Epidemic Update: December 2004*, 37.

32. Henry J. Kaiser Family Foundation, "The Global HIV/AIDS Epidemic," HIV/AIDS Policy Fact Sheet, December 2004; available at http://www.kff.org; Internet; accessed 12 December 2004.

33. UNAIDS/WHO, *AIDS Epidemic Update: December 2004*, 36.

34. "AIDS Finally Is Described by the Chinese as Epidemic," *New York Times*, 17 December 2000, NE5; Elisabeth Rosenthal, "China Raises Estimates of H.I.V.-AIDS Cases to 1 Million," *New York Times*, 6 September 2002. International attention had focused on the tens of thousands or more rural villagers who were infected in the early 1990s from blood purchased at collecting centers that did not follow blood donation safety procedures. UNAIDS, *Report on the Global HIV/AIDS Epidemic, 2002*, 29.

35. UNAIDS/WHO, *AIDS Epidemic Update: December 2004*, 37.

36. Ibid.

37. Ibid., 42.

38. Ibid., 37; C. Shengli, Z. Shikun, and S. B. Westley, "HIV/AIDS Awareness Is Improving in China," *Asia-Pacific Population & Policy* 69 (2004):1–5.

39. UNAIDS, *Report on the Global HIV/AIDS Epidemic, 2002*, 29–30.

40. UNAIDS/WHO, *AIDS Epidemic Update: December 2004*, 37.

41. Ibid., 46.

42. Nicholas Eberstadt, "The Future of AIDS," *Foreign Affairs* 81, no. 6 (2002): 22–45 at 44.

43. UNAIDS/WHO, *AIDS Epidemic Update: December 2002*, 21.

44. UNAIDS/WHO, *AIDS Epidemic Update: December 2004*, 4, 31, 57.

45. UNAIDS, *Report on the Global HIV/AIDS Epidemic, July 2004*; Henry J. Kaiser Family Foundation, "The Global HIV/AIDS Epidemic."

46. UNAIDS/WHO, *AIDS Epidemic Update: December 2004*, 4.

47. Ibid., 57; J. R. P. Marins et al. "Dramatic Improvement in Survival among Adult Brazilian AIDS Patients," *AIDS* 17, no. 11 (2003): 1675–82.

48. UNAIDS/WHO, *AIDS Epidemic Update: December 2004*, 57; N. Gravato, M. G. G. Morell, K. Areco, and C. A. Peres, "Associated Factors to HIV Infection in Commercial Sex Workers in Santos, Sao Paulo, Brazil," Abstract WePeC6162, presented at XV International AIDS Conference, Bangkok, 11–16 July, 2004.

49. UNAIDS/WHO, *AIDS Epidemic Update: December 2004*, 57–58.

50. Ibid., 58; Ministerio de Salud de Argentina, *Boletin sobre el SIDA en la Argentina* 10, no. 22 (October 2003) (Buenos Aires: Ministerio de Salud); M. De los Pando et al., "High Human Immunodeficiency Virus Type 1 Seroprevalence in Men Who Have Sex with Men in Buenos Aires, Argentina: Risk Factors for Infection," *International Journal of Epidemiology* 32 (2003): 735–40.

51. UNAIDS/WHO, *AIDS Epidemic Update: December 2004*, 58.

52. Jo Alarcon et al., "Determinants and Prevalence of HIV Infection in Pregnant Peruvian Women," *AIDS* 17 (2003): 613–18; UNAIDS/WHO, *AIDS Epidemic Update: December 2004*, 58.

53. K. M. Johnson et al., "Sexual Networks of Pregnant Women with and without HIV Infection," *AIDS* 17, no. 4 (2003): 605–12; UNAIDS/WHO, *AIDS Epidemic Update: December 2004*, 58. Further: "In a general population study in 24 Peruvian cities, 44% of men aged 18 to 29 years said they paid for sex (45% of them did not consistently use condoms with sex workers) and 12% said they had sex with other men (68% of them did not use condoms consistently in those encounters)." 58. See J. Guanira et al., "Second Generation of HIV Surveillance among Men Who Have Sex with Men in Peru during 2002," Abstract WePe6162, presented at the XV International AIDS Conference, Bangkok, 11–16 July 2004.

54. UNAIDS/WHO, *AIDS Epidemic Update: December 2004*, 60.

55. UNAIDS/WHO, *AIDS Epidemic Update: December 2002*, 21.

56. UNAIDS, *Report on the Global HIV/AIDS Epidemic, 2002*, 36.

57. Ibid., 37.

58. UNAIDS/WHO, *AIDS Epidemic Update: December 2004*, 61. A recent study in Brazil "calculated that median survival was just under five years (58 months) for people diagnosed with AIDS in 1996, while it was only 18 months for those diagnosed in 1995." J. R. P. Marins et al., "Dramatic Improvement in Survival among Adult Brazilian AIDS Patients," *AIDS* 17, no. 11 (2003): 1675–82.

59. UNAIDS/WHO, *AIDS Epidemic Update: December 2004*, 32.

60. Ibid., 32–33.

61. Ibid., 34.

62. Ibid. C. J. Palmer et al., "HIV Prevalence in a Gold Mining Camp in the Ama-

zon Region, Guyana," *Emerging Infectious Diseases* 8, no. 3 (March 2002); available at http://www.cdc.gov/ncidod/eid/vol8no3/01-0261.htm.

63. UNAIDS/WHO, *AIDS Epidemic Update: December 2004*, 34.

64. Ibid., 33. M. A. St. John et al., "Efficacy of Nevirapine Administration on Mother-to-Child Transmission of HIV Using a Modified HIVNET 012 Regimen," *West Indian Medical Journal* 51, Suppl. 3 (2003): 1–87.

65. UNAIDS/WHO, *AIDS Epidemic Update: December 2004*, 47–48. The Russian Federation accounts for about 70% of all HIV infections officially registered in the region. 47.

66. Ibid., 47–48.

67. For example, in 2002 in sub-Saharan Africa, without including any antiretroviral medicine, the annual medical cost of AIDS is estimated at about $30 per person. This is a real challenge when overall annual public health spending is less than $10 per person in most African countries. UNAIDS, *Report on the Global HIV/AIDS Epidemic, 2002*, 50. See also Tina Rosenberg, "How to Solve the World's AIDS Crisis," *New York Times Magazine*, 28 January 2001, 26.

68. For information regarding the Jubilee Debt Campaign, see "Jubilee Research: Supporting Economic Justice Campaigns Worldwide"; available at http://lb.bcentral.com/ex/manage/subscriberprefs.aspx?customerid=25096; Internet; accessed 8 September 2003.

69. UNAIDS, *Report on the Global HIV/AIDS Epidemic—AIDS in a New Millennium, 2000*, 1.

70. UNAIDS, *Report on the Global HIV/AIDS Epidemic, 2002*, 44–59.

71. WHO, "Key Facts from The World Health Report 2004," *The World Health Report 2004: Changing History*, May 2004, Geneva. Another challenging figure from Africa is that it is estimated that in 1999, 5,500 AIDS funerals occurred in Africa every day. Jon D. Fuller and James F. Keenan, "Introduction," in *Catholic Ethicists on HIV/AIDS Prevention*. See WHO, *World Health Report, 1999*, Geneva.

72. UNAIDS, *Report on the Global HIV/AIDS Epidemic, July 2004*.

73. Ibid.

74. Ibid.; Henry J. Kaiser Family Foundation, "The Global HIV/AIDS Epidemic."

75. UNAIDS, *Report on the Global HIV/AIDS Epidemic—AIDS in a New Millennium, 2000*, 1.

76. UNAIDS, *Report on the Global HIV/AIDS Epidemic, 2002*, 83.

77. UNAIDS, *Report on the Global HIV/AIDS Epidemic, 2002*, states that among young people, "most HIV infections occur during, or soon after, adolescence." 83.

78. Ibid., 86.

79. See, for example, Microbicides Development Programme, "Why Do We Need a Microbicide?" available at http://www.mdp.mrc.ac.uk/uhat.html; Internet; accessed 27 May 2005. Non-contraceptive microbicides would allow a woman to conceive while at the same time offering HIV transmission protection. This is still in experimental stages.

80. See, for example, Jorge J. Ferrer, "Needle Exchange in San Juan, Puerto Rico: A Traditional Roman Catholic Casuistic Approach," in *Catholic Ethicists*, 177–91.

81. NIAID, *HIV Infection and AIDS*, 4.

82. WHO, "Key Facts from The World Health Report 2004," *The World Health Report 2004: Changing History*, May 2004.

83. Ibid.

84. UNAIDS, *Report on the Global HIV/AIDS Epidemic, 2002*, 83.

85. Ibid., 142. The declaration makes the following commitments: ". . . by 2003, ensure that national strategies, supported by regional and international strategies, are developed . . . to strengthen health-care systems and address factors affecting the provision of HIV-related drugs, including antiretroviral drugs, inter alia, affordability and pricing, including differential pricing, and technical and health-care system capacity. . . ." *United Nations General Assembly Special Session on HIV/AIDS*, June 2001, New York, para. 55.

86. WHO, "Key Facts from The World Health Report 2004."

87. UNAIDS, *Report on the Global HIV/AIDS Epidemic, 2002*, 146.

88. Ibid., 148. For example, Cipla Ltd., an Indian generics manufacturer, contracted with the Nigerian Health Ministry to sell combination antiretroviral therapy for $350 per client per year.

89. UNAIDS/WHO, *AIDS Epidemic Update: December 2002*, 23.

90. WHO, "Key Facts from The World Health Report 2004," *The World Health Report 2004: Changing History*, May 2004, Geneva.

91. UNAIDS, *Report on the Global HIV/AIDS Epidemic, 2002*, 147. Two NGOs that have prioritized advocacy for antiretrovirals for low- and middle-income countries include OXFAM and Médecins Sans Frontières.

92. See Tina Rosenberg, "How to Solve the World's AIDS Crisis" and Johanna McGreary, "Paying for AIDS Cocktails: Who Should Pick Up the Tab for the Third World?" *Time*, 12 February 2001, 54.

93. Henry J. Kaiser Family Foundation. "The Global HIV/AIDS Epidemic."

94. U.S. Congress, H.R. 4818, Consolidated Appropriation, FY2005 and conference report (H.R. 108–792), includes 83% rescission; Henry J. Kaiser Family Foundation, "The Global HIV/AIDS Epidemic."

95. As I will develop it, especially in the first two chapters, the term "poverty" encompasses the economic and structural inequalities and injustices that result in various forms of poverty. So intertwined is poverty with various forms of inequality and injustice that I do not want to privilege one term over another. Therefore, while I will use "poverty" as the overarching term; the other terms will also be used in discussions of various dimensions of this second foundational contributor to HIV/AIDS.

96. Found in Kevin Kelly, "Conclusion: A Moral Theologian Faces the New Millennium in a Time of AIDS," in *Catholic Ethicists*, 325. See also Teresa Okure, SHCJ, "HIV and Women: Gender Issues, Culture and Church," paper presented at the Consultation on HIV/AIDS, Bertoni Centre, Pretoria, April 1999, 1–13.

97. Summarized in Kelly, "Conclusion," 325.

98. Ibid.

99. Ibid. Theologian Denise M. Ackermann adds a third "virus," that of denial. She is not referring to individual denial by people who refuse to be tested for the virus because they find the prospect of infection to be too shattering. Ackermann writes that "more pernicious than individual denial has been the denial by the South African state that its citizens are trapped in a pandemic." Until April 2002 President Mbeki refused to acknowledge scientific facts regarding HIV/AIDS and refused virtually free treatment to prevent the transmission of the virus from HIV-infected pregnant women to their newborns. Denise M. Ackermann, "'Deep in the Flesh':

Women, Bodies and HIV/AIDS: Feminist Ethical Perspective" (manuscript sent from South Africa). See also Ackermann, "Reconciliation as Embodied Change: A South African Perspective." *Proceedings of the Catholic Theological Society of America* 59 (2004):50–67.

100. Paul Farmer, "Women, Poverty, and AIDS," in *Women, Poverty, and AIDS: Sex, Drugs and Structural Violence*, eds. Paul Farmer, Maureen Connors, and Janie Simmons (Monroe, ME: Common Courage Press, 1996), 3–38.

101. Lisa Sowle Cahill, "AIDS, Justice, and the Common Good," in *Catholic Ethicists on HIV/AIDS Prevention*, ed. James F. Keenan, assisted by Jon D. Fuller, Lisa Sowle Cahill, and Kevin Kelly (New York: Continuum, 2000), 284.

102. Ibid. Richard G. Parker, "Empowerment, Community Mobilization, and Social Change in the Face of HIV/AIDS," paper presented at the XI International Conference on AIDS, Vancouver, July 1996, 6–7.

103. UNAIDS/WHO, *AIDS Epidemic Update: December 2002*, 19.

104. Ibid., 33.

105. See, for example, UNAIDS, *Gender and HIV/AIDS: Taking Stock of Research and Programmes*, 1999.

106. UNAIDS, "Fact Sheets—Men Make a Difference," 1; available at http://www.unaids.org/fact_sheets/files/WAC_Eng.html; Internet; accessed 15 November 2000.

107. Ibid., 2.

108. Nafis Sadik, "Gender Dimensions of HIV/AIDS: A Key Challenge to Rural Development," United Nations, New York, 30 April 2004, 6; available at http://www.un.org/esa/coordination/ecosoc/hl2003/RT2%20Sadik.pdf; Internet; accessed 30 June 2004.

109. "Wife-Beating in Zambia a 'Natural Consequence,'" *Mail & Guardian online*, 17 September 2004; available at http://www.mg.co.za/Content/13.asp?ao= 24385; Internet; accessed 17 September 2004; "Zambia Demographic and Health Survey, 2001–2002." Calverton, Maryland: Central Statistics Office and Macro International Inc., February 2003. See also Joanna Bourke-Martignoni, "Violence against Women in Zambia," report prepared for the Committee on the Elimination of Discrimination against Women, available at http://www.omct/pdf/vaw/zambi-aeng2002.pdf; Internet; accessed 7 September 2004.

110. UNAIDS/WHO, *AIDS Epidemic Update: December 2004*, 10; UNAIDS, "Women and AIDS—A Growing Challenge," Fact Sheet; available at http://www.unaids.org/html/pub/publications/fact-sheets04/FS_Women_en_pdf; Internet; accessed 9 December 2004.

111. UNAIDS, "Have You Heard Me Today? World AIDS Campaign on Women and Girls;" available at http://www.unaids.org/wac2004/index_en.htm; Internet; accessed 27 December 2004.

112. Peter Piot, "Message on the Occasion of World AIDS Day"; available at http://www.unaids.org/html/pub/media/speeches02/SP_Piot_WAD2004_01Dec04_ en_pdf; Internet; accessed 27 December 2004.

113. UNAIDS, *Report on the Global HIV/AIDS Epidemic, 2002*, 16.

114. The 2001 Declaration of Commitment states that by 2003 there will be in place in "all countries strategies, policies and programmes that identify and begin to address those factors that make individuals particularly vulnerable to HIV infection, including underdevelopment, economic insecurity, poverty, lack of empower-

ment of women, lack of education, social exclusion, illiteracy, discrimination, lack of information and/or commodities for self-protection, all types of sexual exploitation of women, girls and boys, including for commercial reasons. . . ." United Nations General Assembly Special Session on HIV/AIDS, June 2001, New York, para. 62.

115. UNAIDS, *Report on the Global HIV/AIDS Epidemic, 2002*, 61.

116. See, for example, Pope Paul VI, "Encyclical Letter on the Regulation of Births," *Humanae Vitae*, 25 July 1968. In *Vatican Council II: More Postconciliar Documents* (English edition), ed. Austin Flannery (Grand Rapids, MI: Eerdmans, 1982); Pope John Paul II, *The Theology of the Body: Human Love in the Divine Plan* (Boston, MA: Pauline Books, 1997); United States Catholic Council of Bishops (USCCB), *Human Sexuality: A Catholic Perspective for Education and Lifelong Learning* (Washington, D.C.: USCC, 1997).

117. Fuller and Keenan, "Introduction," 22; see also "Reaction to AIDS Statement," *Origins* 17.28 (1987): 489–93; "Continued Reaction to AIDS Statement," *Origins* 17.30 (1988): 516–22; "Cardinal Ratzinger's Letter on AIDS Document," *Origins* 18.8 (1988): 117–21. Others respond that information about appropriate use of condoms does not increase the rate of sexual intercourse. See, for example, Sally Guttmacher, Lisa Lieberman, and David Ward, "Does Access to Condoms Influence Adolescent Sexual Behavior?" *The AIDS Reader* 8 (November/December 1998): 201–205, 209; Deborah E. Sellers, Sarah A. McGraw, and John B. McKinlay, "Does the Promotion and Distribution of Condoms Increase Teen Sexual Activity? Evidence from an HIV Prevention Program for Latino Youth," *American Journal of Public Health* 84 (December 1994): 1952–59; Douglas Kirby, Nancy D. Brener, Ron Harrist, et al., "The Impact of Condom Distribution in Seattle Schools on Sexual Behavior and Condom Use," *American Journal of Public Health* 89 (February 1999): 182–87.

118. See, for example, James Keenan, "Prophylactics, Toleration and Cooperation: Contemporary Moral Problems and Traditional Principles," *International Philosophical Quarterly* 28 (1988): 201–20; Jon Fuller, *AIDS and the Church: A Stimulus to Our Theologizing*, lecture given at Weston Jesuit School of Theology, Boston, MA, 12 March 1991; Jon Fuller, "AIDS Prevention: A Challenge to the Catholic Moral Tradition," *America* 175 (28 December 1996): 13–20; Jon Fuller and James Keenan, "Condoms, Catholics and HIV/AIDS Prevention," *The Furrow* 52, no. 9 (Sept. 2001): 459–67.

119. See, for example, Jon D. Fuller and James F. Keenan, "Church Politics and HIV Prevention: Why Is the Condom Question So Significant and So Neuralgic?" in *Between Poetry and Politics: Essays in Honour of Enda McDonagh*, eds. Barbara Fitzgerald and Linda Hogan (Dublin: Columba Press, 2003). Condoms can break; they can degrade without proper storage or with inappropriate (petroleum-based) lubricants; condoms can be improperly manufactured and improperly used.

120. Fuller and Keenan, "Church Politics and HIV Prevention." The authors cite the National Institute of Allergy and Infectious Diseases (NIAID) STD Report. They further write: "As that meta-analysis noted, it must first be appreciated that HIV is a very inefficiently transmitted infection when compared with other common sexually transmitted diseases. For example, a single exposure to gonorrhea causes infection in 60%–80% of women. In contrast, after a single exposure to HIV, only 0.1%–0.2% of women become infected. The study found that use of condoms reduces the already low transmission rate of HIV by 85%. If one applied these data to 10,000 persons being exposed to HIV during sexual intercourse over a period of one year, in

the absence of condoms 670 would become infected, while that number would be reduced to 90 if condoms were used consistently and correctly" (5). A challenge is that women often lack any control over whether a male partner or husband uses the prophylactic. Research on non-contraceptive microbicides may offer promise in years to come for some protection against HIV while still allowing for conception.

121. For an explanation of material cooperation, see James F. Keenan, "Prophylactics, Toleration and Cooperation"; James F. Keenan and Thomas Kopfensteiner, "The Principle of Material Cooperation," *Health Progress* 76.3 (April 1995): 23–27. A brief explanation of the principle of cooperation is found in the appendix of the 1995 Ethical and Religious Directives for Catholic Health Care Services:

> The principles governing cooperation differentiate the action of the wrongdoer from the action of the cooperator through two major distinctions. The first is between formal and material cooperation. If the cooperator intends the object of the wrongdoer's activity, then the cooperation is formal and, therefore, morally wrong. Since intention is not simply an explicit act of the will, formal cooperation can also be implicit. Implicit formal cooperation is attributed when, even though the cooperator denies intending the wrongdoer's object, no other explanation can distinguish the cooperator's object from the wrongdoer's object. If the cooperator does not intend the object of the wrongdoer's activity, the cooperation is material and can be morally licit.
>
> The second distinction deals with the object of the action and is expressed by immediate and mediate material cooperation. Material cooperation is immediate when the object of the cooperator is the same as the object of the wrongdoer. Immediate material cooperation is wrong, except in some instances of duress. The matter of duress distinguishes immediate material cooperation from implicit formal cooperation. But immediate material cooperation—without duress—is equivalent to implicit formal cooperation and, therefore, is morally wrong. When the object for the cooperator's action remains distinguishable from that of the wrongdoer's, material cooperation is mediate and can be morally licit.
>
> Moral theologians recommend two other considerations for the proper evaluation of material cooperation. First, the object of material cooperation should be as distant as possible from the wrongdoer's act. Second, any act of material cooperation requires a proportionately grave reason.
>
> Prudence guides those involved in cooperation to estimate the questions of intention, duress, distance, necessity and gravity. In making a judgment about cooperation, it is essential that the possibility of scandal should be eliminated. Appropriate consideration should also be given to the church's prophetic responsibility. [NCCB, "Ethical and Religious Directives for Catholic Health Care Services," *Origins* (December 15, 1994): 449–62.]

122. Roger Burggraeve uses an ethics of mercy to discuss HIV prevention measures for young people. See "From Responsible to Meaningful Sexuality: An Ethics of Growth as an Ethics of Mercy for Young People in this Era of AIDS" in *Catholic Ethicists*, 303–16; "Une Ethique de Miséricorde," *Lumen Vitae: Revue internationale de catéchèse et de pastorale* 49 (September 1994): 281–96; "Prohibition and Taste: The Bipolarity in Christian Ethics," *Ethical Perspectives* 1, no. 3 (1994): 130–44.

123. USCC Administrative Board, *The Many Faces of AIDS: A Gospel Response* (Washington, DC: USCC, Inc., November 1987); National Conference of Catholic

Bishops, *Called to Compassion and Responsibility: A Response to the HIV/AIDS Crisis* (Washington, DC: USCC, Inc., November 1989).

124. As head of the Congregation for the Doctrine of the Faith, Cardinal Joseph Ratzinger wrote to the U.S. bishops that condoms are not an appropriate response to HIV prevention. (See "Cardinal Ratzinger's Letter on AIDS Document," *Origins* 18.8 [1988]: 117–121.) On June 10, 2005 Pope Benedict XVI told bishops from southern Africa on an "ad limina" visit to the Vatican that following the church's teaching of fidelity and chastity "has proven to be the only fail-safe way to prevent the spread of HIV/AIDS." Catholic News Service, available at http://www.catholicnews.com/data/briefs/cns/20050610.htm; Internet; accessed 14 June 2005.

Still, Cardinals Georges Cottier, Godfried Danneels, Cormac Murphy-O'Connor, and Javier Lozano Barragan have voiced their support for the use of prophylactics to limit the spread of AIDS. On January 30, 2005, *The Tablet* reported that Cardinal Cottier, the theologian whom Pope John Paul II named as cardinal and as Head of the Papal household: "told the Italian news agency Apcom last week that the use of condoms was 'legitimate' to save lives in the poorest parts of Africa and Asia where the AIDS pandemic has been catastrophic. He argued that condoms should be tolerated as a 'lesser evil' in instances where the ideals of abstinence and fidelity are simply not realistic.

"Cardinal Cottier reiterated the Church's official line that condoms should not be used as contraceptives, could encourage immoral sexual conduct, and were not the best way to stop the spread of HIV. However, he went on to say the commandment 'Thou shalt not kill' should be considered in cases where sexual activity involves a partner who is HIV positive. 'The virus is transmitted during a sexual act; so at the same time as bringing life there is also a risk of transmitting death,' he said" (*The Tablet*, 5 February 2005, available at http://www.thetablet.co.uk/cgi-bin/citw.cgi/past-00216; accessed 14 June 2005.) The Cardinal here noted that he was giving his own personal opinion and not speaking for the Holy See.

Cardinal Danneels, the archbishop of Brussels, has stated that "If a person infected with HIV has decided not to respect abstinence, then he has to protect his partner and he can do that—in this case—by using a condom." To do otherwise, he said, would be "to break the Fifth Commandment," that you shall not kill (*The Tablet*, 3 July 2004, available at http://www.cardinalrating.com/cardinal_22__article_108.htm; accessed 14 June 2005).

Cardinal Murphy-O'Connor, archbishop of Westminster, England, supported Cardinal Danneels's position. (See "More Tea, Cardinal?" *The Independent*, 26 July 2004, available at http://www.cardinalrating.com/cardinal_65__article_1357.htm; accessed 14 June 2005.)

Cardinal Barragan, president of the Pontifical Council for Health and Pastoral Care, on World AIDS Day 2003, while stressing the importance of programs focusing on abstinence and fidelity, has "condoned the use of condoms in the limited situation where a woman cannot refuse her HIV-positive husband's sexual advances" (Human Rights Watch, December 2004, available at http://hrw.org/backgrounder/hivaids/condoms1204/3.htm#_ftn38; accessed 14 June 2005).

See, also, Craig Whitney, "French Bishop Supports Some Use of Condoms to Prevent AIDS," *New York Times*, 13 February 1996, 5; Pamela Schaeffer, "Condoms Tolerated to Avoid AIDS, French Bishops Say," *National Catholic Reporter*, 23 February 1996, 9; "Caution Greets AIDS Statement by French Bishops," *The Tablet*, 24 February 1996, 256–57; "Church Leaders Mix Condoms and Caveats," *National*

Catholic Reporter, 15 March 1996. See also "Dutch Cardinal Says Condoms OK When Spouse Has AIDS," *Catholic News Service*, 16 February 1996; "Vienna Archbishop Says Condoms Morally Acceptable to Fight AIDS," *Catholic News Service*, 3 April 1996; Robert Vitillo, "HIV/AIDS Prevention Education: A Special Concern for the Church," presentation for discussion at Caritas International, CAFOD Theological Consultation on HIV/AIDS, Pretoria, South Africa, 14 April 1998). And from the German bishops conference: "before the deadly menace which the AIDS virus effectively represents, it is necessary to do everything to avoid contamination . . . The information must be complete, broad-based and honest, without ceasing to be balanced. It must not become a disguised invitation to sexual license." *La Documentation Catholique* no. 2176 (1998):191–95. See also Most Reverend Anthony M. Pilla, "Statement on Developing an Approach by the Church to AIDS Education," *Origins* 16 (1987): 692–93. The more recent and important Southern African Bishops' debate regarding prophylactic use can be found in Fuller and Keenan, "Church Politics and HIV Prevention"; "South African Bishops to Discuss AIDS, Condom Use," *Catholic News Service*, 11 July 2001; Southern African Bishops' Conference, "A Message of Hope from the Catholic Bishops to the People of God in South African, Botswana and Swaziland," 30 July 2001; "The Church and Condoms," *The Southern Cross*, 10 December 2002, 4; "The Condom Debate," editorial in *The Southern Cross*, 18 July 2001. An overview of this debate among the bishops of South Africa is in Fuller and Keenan, "Church Politics and HIV Prevention."

125. For a theological discussion of needle exchange programs, see, for example, Ferrer, "Needle Exchange in San Juan, Puerto Rico," 177–91; Jon Fuller, "Needle Exchange: Saving Lives," *America* 179 (18–25 July 1998): 8–11.

126. Enda McDonagh, "The Reign of God: Signposts for Catholic Moral Theology," in *Catholic Ethicists*, 317–23.

127. Kevin T. Kelly, *New Directions in Sexual Ethics: Moral Theology and the Challenge of AIDS* (London: Geoffrey Chapman, 1998).

2. Toward a Fundamental Theological Anthropology

1. This is not to say that theology or the Catholic Church has yet fully lived out such a response. However, there are helpful resources in the tradition. The Church is also a dynamic institution, always growing and deepening in its integration of the signs of the times, the tradition, and the experiences of its people, all in service of the people of God.

2. Mary Ann Hinsdale, "Heeding the Voices: An Historical Overview," in *In The Embrace of God: Feminist Approaches to Theological Anthropology*, ed. Ann O'Hara Graff (Maryknoll, NY: Orbis Books, 1995), 22.

3. Janet K. Ruffing, "Anthropology, Theological," in *The New Dictionary of Catholic Spirituality*, ed. Michael Downey (Collegeville, MN: Liturgical Press, 1993), 47.

4. Hinsdale, "Heeding the Voices," 22.

5. Conversely, HIV/AIDS affects theology and helps us to mine its resources and to respond to its growing edges.

6. In the opening pages of a collection of essays on the mystical-political dimensions of Christianity, Metz offers a brief biographical itinerary of his theology. In trying to "show how the itinerary of political theology has been a reflection of my life," Metz relates his experience as a sixteen-year-old near the end of World War II, who

was forced into the army and sent to the front with over a hundred in his company, most of whom were also very young. Carrying a message to battalion headquarters one evening, he passed destroyed, burning villages. On his return the next morning he found the dead bodies of his entire company. "I could see only dead and empty faces, where the day before I had shared childhood fears and youthful laughter. I remembered nothing but a wordless cry. Thus I see myself to this very day, and behind this memory all my childhood dreams crumble away." Johann Baptist Metz, *A Passion for God: The Mystical-Political Dimension of Christianity*, ed. and trans. J. Matthew Ashley (New York: Paulist Press, 1998), 1–2.

7. Metz is helpful because even if prophylactics are condoned, supported, or advocated by political or ecclesial leaders, gender inequality and social injustice will still exist. Only a conversion of mind and heart will in the end change the practices that foundationally affect AIDS. Furthermore, although Metz's sympathies are similar to those of liberation theology, he primarily addresses and engages the First World. And Metz acknowledges that efforts on behalf of justice may take one form for citizens of the First World and another form for Third World citizens. The goals may be similar, but the contexts are different.

8. Johann Baptist Metz, *Faith in History and Society: Toward a Practical Fundamental Theology*, trans. David Smith (New York: Seabury Press, 1980), 102.

9. According to Ashley, Metz is not seeking an exhaustive theological anthropology, "but rather intends only to uncover the basic categories in terms of which the broader project—determining humans' constitutive depth-relation to God—can be worked out." J. Matthew Ashley, *Interruptions: Mysticism, Politics, and Theology in the Work of Johann Baptist Metz* (Notre Dame, IN: University of Notre Dame Press, 1998), 148.

10. Mary Catherine Hilkert, in her excellent work, *Naming Grace: Preaching and the Sacramental Imagination* (New York: Continuum, 1997), writes, "the human struggle with suffering is ultimately a spiritual crisis." 115.

11. Suffering here does not include existential suffering or angst. The suffering mentioned above is a response to concrete, oppressive, and debilitating circumstances. This suffering is *not*, in Jon Sobrino's words, "from the (apparently) universal perspective of the metaphysical suffering characterizing all finite being." Jon Sobrino, *The Principle of Mercy: Taking the Crucified People from the Cross* (Maryknoll, NY: Orbis Books, 1994), 33.

12. These voices include, among others, Gustavo Gutiérrez, Jon Sobrino, and Ignatio Ellacuría from liberation theology; Margaret Farley, Lisa Cahill, Ivone Gebara, Denise Ackermann, and Barbara Hilkert Andolsen from feminist theology; Teresa Okure and Mercy Amba Oduyoye from African theology; and Johann B. Metz from political theology.

13. Edward Schillebeeckx, *Christ: The Experience of Jesus as Lord*, trans. John Bowden (New York: Crossroad, 1981), 650.

14. Patricia McAuliffe, *Fundamental Ethics: A Liberationist Approach* (Washington, DC: Georgetown University Press, 1993), ix.

15. M. Shawn Copeland, "'Wading Through Many Sorrows': Toward a Theology of Suffering in Womanist Perspective," in *Feminist Ethics and the Catholic Moral Tradition*, eds. Charles E. Curran, Margaret A. Farley, and Richard A. McCormick (New York: Paulist Press, 1996), 136.

16. Ignacio Ellacuria, "The Crucified People," in *Mysterium Liberationis: Fundamental Concepts of Liberation Theology*, eds. Ignatio Ellacuría and Jon Sobrino (Maryknoll, NY: Orbis Books, 1993), 580.

17. Sobrino, *Principle of Mercy*, 27.

18 Ibid., 30. Sobrino also acknowledges many other causes of massive poverty in the world, including race, sex, and caste. He reminds us that, "to a great extent, those who suffer the indignity and pain of racial, sexual, or caste discrimination also belong to the world of the poor, which sharpens their suffering and makes it all the more difficult for them to liberate themselves from such indignity." 33.

19. Sobrino, *Principle of Mercy*, 32.

20. Metz, "Theology and the University," in *Passion for God*, 134.

21. Ibid., 4.

22. Edward Schillebeeckx, *Christ, the Sacrament of the Encounter with God* (New York: Sheed and Ward, 1963), 818.

23. Metz, *Passion for God*, 196.

24. Ibid., 134.

25. Ashley, *Interruptions*, 157. In the next section, we shall see how Metz's understanding of history is colored by the reality of suffering and resistance, and how this moves him and us to a recognition of one's complicity in the sufferings of the other.

26. While the limits of this book do not allow for the development of an extensive theology of the cross, there are certainly many who are working on or have contributed to this theologically important topic (e.g., Mary Catherine Hilkert, Dietrich Bonhoeffer, Dorothee Soelle).

27. Hilkert, *Naming Grace*, 112. Hilkert offers a brief description of some early understandings of the cross from the resurrection communities to Abelard, Aquinas, and Luther (112–13). Key for us today will also be understanding suffering in parts of the world, the experiences and perspectives of which have not been considered until more recently. Latin American liberation theology has certainly brought in the experience of one part of the Southern Hemisphere. However, Asian and African voices are also essential and need to be further explored. In light of the AIDS pandemic ravaging much of the African continent, listening to these voices is critical to a contemporary understanding of the cross and resurrection.

28. Hilkert, *Naming Grace*, 113. It must also be noted that theories of atonement have been under severe critique and, in light of women's and children's experiences of suffering, have been found especially wanting by feminists. Feminist theologians from various cultures, races, and classes are "grappling with the experience of suffering, the paschal mystery, the compassion of God, and contemporary metaphors for salvation."114. A critical perspective on a later appropriation of Anselm's atonement theory in the tradition can be found in Elizabeth A. Johnson, "Jesus and Salvation," *Proceedings of the Catholic Theological Society of America* 49 (1994): 1–18.

29. Hilkert, *Naming Grace*, 114.

30. Mary Catherine Hilkert, *Speaking with Authority: Catherine of Siena and the Voices of Women Today*, 2001 Madeleva Lecture in Spirituality (New York: Paulist Press, 2001), 119.

31. Ibid., 118.

32. The resurrection is also the precursor of hope, a virtue developed in subsequent chapters.

33. Hilkert, *Naming Grace*, 115.

34. Hilkert, *Speaking with Authority*, 119.

35. Hilkert, *Naming Grace*, 115. This is not to say, however, that all suffering has meaning; some does not. Hilkert acknowledges that "profound experiences of

suffering bring us to the limits of our lives and of the meaning-systems we embrace." *Naming Grace*, 108.

36. Leonardo Boff, *When Theology Listens to the Poor*, trans. Robert R. Barr (San Francisco: Harper & Row, 1988), 120–21.

37. Sobrino, *Principle of Mercy*, 10.

38. Hilkert, *Naming Grace*, 114.

39. Luke 4:18–19; Isaiah 61:1–2.

40. Edward Schillebeeckx, *Jesus: An Experiment in Christology*, trans. Hubert Hoskins (New York: Seabury Press, 1979), 178.

41. Sobrino, *Principle of Mercy*, 1–11.

42. Ashley, *Interruptions*, 127. Interestingly, in terms of the book of Job, J. David Pleins, in his essay " 'Why Do You Hide Your Face?' Divine Silence and Speech in the Book of Job," *Interpretation* 48 (July 1994), writes of God's silence as a stance of listening. 229–240, at 230. Cited in Keenan, "Suffering and the Christian Tradition," *The Yale Journal for Humanities in Medicine*, 4. available at http://info.med. yale.edu/intmed/hummed/yjhm/spirit/suffering/jkeenanprint.htm; Internet; accessed 10 September 2003.

43. Ashley, *Interruptions*, 126.

44. Walter Brueggemann also explicitly connects Israel's experience of radical absence and anguish, as found in the Psalms. Hilkert, *Naming Grace*, 82.

45. Hilkert, *Naming Grace*, 83.

46. The *Oxford American Dictionary* defines "sass" as impudence or impertinent speech, and the *Random House Dictionary of the English Language* defines "sass" as impudent or disrespectful back talk.

47. Copeland, "Wading Through Many Sorrows," 136–63.

48. Ibid., 152–53, quoting Joanne M. Braxton, *Black Women Writing Autobiography: A Tradition within a Tradition* (Philadelphia: Temple University Press, 1988).

49. Hilkert, *Speaking with Authority*, 122. Hilkert is summarizing Copeland.

50. Copeland, "Wading Through Many Sorrows," 149.

51. Ibid., 150.

52. An example of sass on a large scale occurred at the beginning of this millennium when South Africa threatened to disregard U.S. pressures and pharmaceutical patent laws because drug treatment costs were prohibitive for most of its population. Brazil's efforts to make its drugs available to all of its people with HIV/AIDS and its ability to demonstrate that people can follow a regimen of medicine even under some challenging situations was another example of sass.

53. Ashley, *Interruptions*, 147.

54. "Can" implies intentionality and choice in our perception and action in this regard, especially on the part of North Americans.

55. Ashley, *Interruptions*, 147. Ashley explains this well as he analyzes Metz's fourth chapter of *Faith in History and Society*: "Concept of a Political Theology as a Practical Fundamental Theology" (142–47).

56. Engelbert Mveng, "Impoverishment and Liberation: A Theological Approach for Africa and the Third World," in *Paths of African Theology*, ed. Rosino Gibellini, (Maryknoll, NY: Orbis Books, 1994), 156–58.

57. Ibid., 156.

58. Ibid., 156. In relationship to our discussion of embeddedness in history and society, Mveng writes: "When persons are deprived not only of goods and possessions of a material, spiritual, moral, intellectual, cultural, or sociological order, but

of everything that makes up the foundation of their being-in-the-world and the specificity of their 'ipseity' as individual, society, and history—when persons are bereft of their identity, their dignity, their freedom, their thought, their history, their language, their faith universe, and their basic creativity, deprived of all their ways of living and existing—they sink into a kind of poverty which no longer concerns only exterior or interior goods or possessions but strikes at the very being, essence, and dignity of the human person. It is this poverty that we call anthropological poverty" (156). This has profound ramifications for an understanding of the person in history.

59. Ibid., 157.

60. Ibid., 159.

61. Ibid.

62. Ibid., 160, 164.

63. Ibid., 165.

64. The message is similar to Gutiérrez's claim that the poor are breaking into history: "the poor are freeing themselves from oppressive ideologies and are anticipating new ways of being human." Rebecca Chopp, *The Praxis of Suffering: An Interpretation of Liberation and Political Theologies* (Maryknoll, NY: Orbis Books, 1986), 145.

65. Jean-Marc Ela, "Christianity and Liberation in Africa," in *Paths of African Theology*, 137.

66. Ibid.

67. Ibid., 146.

68. Ibid.

69. Ibid., 137; Luke 10:30–32 NAB.

70 Ela, "Christianity and Liberation," 139. He cites internal corruption and an elite in Africa who are also perpetuating an abusive system of power.

71. Ibid., 138. He writes: "What meaning can faith have in churches that seek to be liberated without sharing the peoples' battles with the forces of oppression assaulting their dignity?"

72. Ibid., 143.

73. Ibid.

74. Cahill writes: "the primary cause of the spread of this horrendous disease is poverty. Related barriers to AIDS prevention are racism; the low status of women; and an exploitive global economic system, which influences marketing of medical resources." "AIDS, Justice and the Common Good," in *Catholic Ethicists on HIV/ AIDS Prevention*, ed. James F. Keenan, assisted by Jon D. Fuller, Lisa Sowle Cahill, and Kevin Kelly (New York: Continuum, 2000), 282.

75. Cahill states: "Key elements in the Catholic vision of social justice and the common good are the dignity of the human person; the comprehensive common good of society; the need for affirmative action toward those currently most excluded from participation in the common good (preferential option for the poor); the reality of structural sin; and the principle of subsidiarity, designating the reciprocal functions of local, national, and international structures of justice." Cahill, "AIDS, Justice and the Common Good," 286. An important resource on the common good is David Hollenbach, *The Common Good and Christian Ethics* (Cambridge: Cambridge University Press, 2002). See also Brian Stiltner, *Religion and the Common Good: Catholic Contributions to Building Community in a Liberal Society* (Lanham, MD: Rowman & Littlefield, 1999).

76. Cahill, "AIDS, Justice and the Common Good," 282.

77. Cahill cites Mark Harrington, a representative of an AIDS action group in New York City: "When we talk about the North-South gap, we must remember that the South includes Mississippi, and it includes the South Bronx." Cahill, "AIDS, Justice and the Common Good," 285.

78. Cahill, "AIDS, Justice and the Common Good," 287–88.

79. Ibid., 288. In *Peace on Earth*, John XXIII writes that the "common good touches the whole man, the needs both of his body and of his soul . . . the common good of all embraces the sum total of those conditions of social living whereby men are enabled to achieve their own integral perfection more fully and more easily." *Pacem in Terris*, in *Catholic Social Thought: The Documentary Heritage*, eds. David J. O'Brien and Thomas A. Shannon (Maryknoll, NY: Orbis Books, 1992), nos. 57, 58.

80. Ivone Gebara, "Women Doing Theology in Latin America," in *Liberation Theology: An Introductory Reader*, eds. Curt Cardorette, Marie Giblin, Marilyn J. Legge, and Mary H. Snyder (Maryknoll, NY: Orbis Books, 1992), 59.

81. Ibid.

82. Luz Beatriz Arellano, "Women's Experience of God in Emerging Spirituality," in *Feminist Theology from the Third World: A Reader*, ed. Ursula King (Maryknoll, NY: Orbis Books, 1994), 323. This is not to deny, however, the need for a hermeneutics of suspicion in the reading of scripture.

83. Arellano, "Women's Experience of God," 323.

84. Ibid., 323. A variety of female authors writing in *Feminist Theology from the Third World* offer this observation.

85. Arellano, "Women's Experience of God," 322.

86. Ibid.

3. Embodied Relational Agent

1. A note of introduction may be helpful here. Since Vatican II, a significant shift in moral theology that flowed from the Council was using the terminology "human person" to replace "human nature." This shift allowed moral decisions to be based on the totality of the person rather than simply on "the finality of bodily structures and functions." Richard Gula, *Reason Informed by Faith: Foundations of Catholic Morality* (New York: Paulist Press, 1989), 63. Gula further writes that the personalistic foundation for morality was laid out in *Gaudium et Spes*, and that Louis Janssens studied this document and affirmed that "human activity must be judged insofar as it refers to the human person integrally and adequately considered." Louis Janssens, "Artificial Insemination: Ethical Considerations," *Louvain Studies* 8 (Spring 1980): 4; in Gula, *Reason Informed by Faith*, 64. In his excellent synthesis of fundamental moral theology, Gula develops Louis Janssens's notion of the human person through an understanding of the person as the image of God and with the fundamental elements of the human person to include the following: "a relational being, an embodied subject, an historical being, and a being fundamentally equal to others but uniquely original," 64. Although all of these elements are essential, for the purpose of this project, I will limit the discussion to three specific areas that need urgent examination in the current situation of AIDS.

2. I am not proposing here a complete or full theology of human sexuality, but am only considering one element of the reality of sexual ethics in the midst of an HIV

pandemic in which coerced sex and infidelity in marriage are unfortunate but significant realities.

3. This is my working definition.

4. Why are these terms so important in discussions of AIDS and moral theology? Because studies continue to show that women and vulnerable populations are more often considered objects that have no ability to make choices and that live in order to survive instead of to thrive. Love often is not seen as important as meeting the needs of an other who may not even desire a committed relationship, but simply uses a partner for his or her own needs and wants. Participation becomes a farce when there are few choices that can be made for full human flourishing. Finally, and most challenging for our current sexual ethics, the person is too often seen without the dynamic capacity for growth—in one's understanding of self, the other, or God; in the body as conduit of love of God, self, and the other; and in deepening levels of commitment. Dynamism appeals to the best in people, offering an attractive message of and to the self and of and to the other.

5. James Keenan cites Stuart Hampshire, who asserts that "the agent has privileged information about the influence that an action could have on the agent's own self." "The Moral Agent: Actions and Normative Decision-Making," in *A Call to Fidelity: On the Moral Theology of Charles E. Curran*, ed. James J. Walter, Timothy E. O'Connell, and Thomas A. Shannon (Washington, DC: Georgetown University Press, 2002), 41. See also Stuart Hampshire, *Thought and Action* (Notre Dame, IN: University of Notre Dame Press, 1983).

6. Margaret Farley distinguishes a feminist notion of freedom and autonomy from the problematic Kantian autonomy, which is more disembodied and nonrelational. Margaret Farley, "A Feminist Version of Respect for Persons," in *Feminist Ethics and the Catholic Moral Tradition* (Mahwah, NJ: Paulist Press, 1996), 169.

7. Gula, *Reason Informed by Faith*, 68. Citing Aquinas, Gula writes: "The Catholic tradition has been clear that we cannot speak of morality in any true sense apart from human persons who are able to act knowingly and willingly" (cf. *Summa Theologiae*, I–II, prologue).

8. Participation also has as an aim the removal of coercive elements from decision-making.

9. Farley, "A Feminist Version," 178.

10. Kevin Kelly discusses this in several sections of *New Directions in Sexual Ethics: Moral Theology and the Challenge of AIDS* (London: Geoffrey Chapman, 1998), 27–39, with special emphasis on these capacities.

11. Farley, "A Feminist Version," 179.

12. I recognize the reality of evil, bad intentions, and wrong acts. They are certainly found in the inequalities, structural injustices, and poverty that assail so much of our world and promote the spread of HIV/AIDS. However, the constructive element of dynamism is to allow for sin and failure to love while at the same time working for good. This is a positive anthropology.

13. The dynamic nature of the agent is essential for constructing a positive sexual ethics rooted in the person's reality.

14. Roberto S. Goizueta, *Caminemos con Jesus: Toward a Hispanic/Latino Theology of Accompaniment* (Maryknoll, NY: Orbis Books, 1995), 64.

15. Ibid., 50.

16. Ibid., 52.

17. Ibid., 66.

18. Goizueta writes that the Trinity is the theological symbol for the "intrinsically and constitutively communal character of God." Goizueta, *Caminemos*, 66.

19. Mercy Amba Oduyoye, *Hearing and Knowing: Theological Reflections on Christianity in Africa* (Maryknoll, NY: Orbis Books, 1986), 140. Theologians such as Denis Edwards, among others, also connect well ecological theology and Trinity. See, for example, Denis Edwards. *Breath of Life: A Theology of the Creator Spirit* (Maryknoll, NY: Orbis Books, 2004).

20. Farley defines agape as a full mutuality marked by equality between the sexes, according to Barbara Hilkert Andolsen, "Agape in Feminist Ethics," *Journal of Religious Ethics* 9.1 (Spring 1981): 77.

21. Margaret Farley, "New Patterns of Relationship: Beginnings of a Moral Revolution," in *Introduction to Christian Ethics: A Reader*, ed. Ronald P. Hamel and Kenneth R. Himes (New York: Paulist Press, 1989), 74. Farley also begins offering alternatives to the traditionally masculine images of the Trinity by utilizing the resources of biology to consider the active role of women in reproduction through images such as mother and father. Hilkert Andolsen's article, "Agape in Feminist Ethics," is seminal in offering a useful feminist critique of agape and an exploration of mutuality as the most appropriate image of Christian love.

22. James F. Keenan, "Christian Perspectives on the Human Body," *Theological Studies* 55 (June 1994): 332.

23. See ibid., 340–42. See also Emily Martin, *The Woman in the Body: A Cultural Analysis of Reproduction* (Boston: Beacon, 1987).

24. Keenan, "Christian Perspectives," 341, quoting S. Kay Toombs, "Illness and the Paradigm of Lived Body," *Theoretical Medicine* 9 (1988): 201–26, at 201.

25. Keenan, "Christian Perspectives," 331–40.

26. Ibid., 344. In addition, Keenan points out recent works, such as Elizabeth A. Johnson, *She Who Is: The Mystery of God in Feminist Theological Discourse* (New York: Crossroad, 1992), which consider the body of Christ to reveal "a fuller understanding of God and a more inclusive understanding of humanity in God's image," 345.

27. Keenan, "Christian Perspectives," 342.

28. Margaret A. Farley, "Sources of Sexual Inequality in the History of Christian Thought," *Journal of Religion* (April 1976): 163–64.

29. Ibid., 164–69.

30. Farley here considers again the nature of the Trinity as a relationship of generativity and mutuality. She helpfully reminds us that "the model of relationship which is revealed in the Trinitarian life is clearly a model of mutuality, equality, infinite reciprocity, and not a model of hierarchy and subordination. The struggle of Trinitarian theology through the centuries to deny any subordination of the second person to the first may be well served by adding the image of masculine-feminine polarity to past images of fatherhood and sonship." "Sources of Sexual Inequality," 174. Furthermore, Farley applauds women who take their own experiences seriously and insist that Christian theology take them seriously as well, for it is "a move to challenge both men and women to understand their sexual and personal identity as incarnational, to come finally to an understanding of equality and mutuality which does not pay the price of alienation from the embodiment which is part of human nature." "Sources of Sexual Inequality," 175.

31. See, for example, John Bradshaw, *Bradshaw on the Family: A New Way of Creating Self-Esteem*, rev. ed. (Deerfield Beach, FL: Health Communications, Inc., 1996).

32. Patricia Jung, "Sanctification: An Interpretation in Light of Embodiment," *Journal of Religious Ethics* 11 (1983): 75–94, is a particularly helpful resource in situating the emotions with virtues that affect the whole embodied person. See also Paul Lauritzen, "Emotions and Religious Ethics," *Journal of Religious Ethics* 16 (1988): 307–24, and James F. Keenan, "Dualism in Medicine, Christian Theology, and the Aging," *Journal of Religion and Health* 35 (1996): 3–46.

33. Elaine Scarry, *The Body in Pain: The Making and Unmaking of the World* (New York: Oxford University Press, 1985), 27–59, at 49.

34. In Keenan, "Christian Perspectives," 344.

35. The use of one's voice also requires that persons are actually *listened to and heard.*

36. In this section I presume that we are all sexual beings, all endowed with sexuality. My focus is more closely on what being sexual means in terms of our bodies in relationship.

37. Fran Ferder and John Heagle, *Tender Fires: The Spiritual Promise of Sexuality* (New York: Crossroad, 2002), 29.

38. Kelly, *New Directions*, 148.

39. I am using the terms "genital intercourse" and "sexual intercourse" interchangeably.

40. Christine Gudorf, in *Body, Sex, and Pleasure: Reconstructing Christian Sexual Ethics* (Cleveland: Pilgrim Press, 1994), discusses the pleasurable aspects of physical sexual intimacy, for each person and for both people. Moreover, pleasure does not mean that every single act of sexual intercourse will be pleasurable for each person. There are times when genital intercourse is more pleasurable for one person than the other, but this again is where the vision of the entire relationship as continually deepening intimacy is key.

41. A newer term, "genitality" is used to specify biological, physical, or genital sexuality. Vincent J. Genovesi, *In Pursuit of Love: Catholic Morality and Human Sexuality*, 2nd ed. (Collegeville, MN: Liturgical Press, 1996), 132; cited in Ferder and Heagle, *Tender Fires*, 30.

42. Family life is yet another crucial element of intimacy and relationship. Although the limits of this project preclude a focused discussion on the family, I clearly acknowledge its importance in discussions of HIV/AIDS today. Two important recent works to consider in terms of family and theology include Lisa Sowle Cahill, *Sex, Gender and Christian Ethics* (Cambridge: Cambridge University Press, 1996), and "Marriage: Developments in Catholic Theology and Ethics," *Theological Studies* 64 (2003): 78–105.

43. Kelly, *New Directions*, 148.

44. One challenge I have tried to consider is whether some of the elements of the sexual expressions of the body for the embodied relational agent might be considered unhelpful outside a U.S. or North American or European context. What would be the response from a conversation with women from various countries and tribal communities in Africa? Can the above elements of a sexual ethics find resonance in a culture other than that of the United States? Although I am unable at this time to complete extensive interviews, conversations with twelve women from parts of Africa, Latin America, and Asia have offered a helpful and illuminating beginning. Their positive responses indicate to me that the context of AIDS is calling for women and men to look further at such sexual ethics and social justice topics.

45. Kelly, *New Directions*, 11. See also Roger Burggraeve, "Une Ethique de mis-

éricorde," *Lumen Vitae: Revue internationale de catéchèse et de pastorale* 49 (September 1994): 281–96, and "Prohibitions and Taste: Bipolarity in Christian Ethics," *Ethical Perspectives* 1 (September 1994): 130–44.

46. I contend that sexual intercourse simply for the purpose of providing basic resources such as food, shelter, and clothing for oneself or for one's family is violent. I also understand that some may contend that there are sex workers who choose, from among other viable options, to be sex workers. However, I have serious reservations about this position.

47. Kelly, *New Directions*, 144. This is directly related to the discussions about *imago Dei* and the Trinity. These theological dimensions continue to offer a rich context for our discussions of theological anthropology.

4. Virtues for a Time of AIDS

1. James F. Keenan, SJ, "Proposing Cardinal Virtues," *Theological Studies* 56 (1995): 711.

2. Lee H. Yearley, "Recent Work on Virtue," *Religious Studies Review* 16 (1990): 2.

3. This is a selective rather than an exhaustive list of virtues essential for responding positively to the reality of HIV/AIDS in the world today. Other virtues such as hospitality and solidarity will be incorporated in a later chapter.

4. James F. Keenan, SJ, "Virtue and Identity," *Concilium* 2 (2000): 69.

5. Antonio Moser and Bernardino Leers, *Moral Theology: Dead Ends and Alternatives*, Theology and Liberation, trans. Paul Burns (Maryknoll, NY: Orbis Books, 1990), 166.

6. Keenan, "Virtue and Identity," 74.

7. Ibid., 74. See also Martha Nussbaum, "Non-Relative Virtues: An Aristotelian Approach," in *Ethical Theory: Character and Virtue*, Midwest Studies in Philosophy 13, ed. P French, T. Uehling, and H. Wettstein (Notre Dame: University of Notre Dame Press, 1988), 32–53.

8. For an extensive bibliography on contemporary writing on virtue ethics, see William C. Spohn, "The Return of Virtue Ethics," *Theological Studies* 53 (1992): 60–75.

9. Alasdair MacIntyre, *After Virtue* (Notre Dame: University of Notre Dame Press, 1988); Stanley Hauerwas, *A Community of Character: Toward a Constructive Christian Social Ethic* (Notre Dame: University of Notre Dame Press, 1981); William C. Spohn, *Go and Do Likewise: Jesus and Ethics* (New York: Continuum, 2000); William Joseph Woodill, *The Fellowship of Life: Virtue Ethics and Orthodox Christianity* (Washington, DC: Georgetown University Press, 1998); Joseph J. Kotva, *The Christian Case for Virtue Ethics* (Washington, DC: Georgetown University Press, 1996); and Moser and Leers, *Moral Theology.*

10. Margaret A. Farley, *Personal Commitments: Beginning, Keeping, Changing* (San Francisco: Harper & Row, 1986); Diana Fritz Cates, *Choosing to Feel: Virtue, Friendship, and Compassion for Friends* (Notre Dame: University of Notre Dame Press, 1997); Marie Vianney Bilgrien, SSND, *Solidarity: A Principle, an Attitude, a Duty? or the Virtue for an Interdependent World?* (New York: Peter Lang Publ., 1999); and Christine D. Pohl, *Making Room: Recovering Hospitality as a Christian Tradition* (Grand Rapids, MI: Eerdmans, 1999).

11. A more recent contribution is Ronaldo Zacharias, SDB, "Virtue Ethics as the Framework for Catholic Sexual Education: Towards the Integration between Being

and Acting in Sexual Education" (STD diss., Weston Jesuit School of Theology, 2002). Zacharias is a Brazilian moral theologian.

12. While the limits of my project do not allow further discussion on this topic, it is important to note that Keenan here works from Thomas Aquinas' cardinal virtues—justice, prudence, fortitude and temperance—and substitutes fortitude and temperance with the virtues of fidelity and self-care. For the reasoning behind Keenan's assertions, see "Proposing Cardinal Virtues."

13. This is especially important for work with ethical issues related to AIDS. For example, many ethicists such as Lisa Sowle Cahill consider AIDS to be a justice issue. I agree. However, I also consider AIDS to be a sexual issue. As a sexual issue, AIDS has implications both for fidelity and for self-care. Keenan's multi-virtue approach is helpful not only in understanding the moral deliberation which is a task of prudence, but also the multi-dimensional approaches necessary for HIV/AIDS prevention.

14. Keenan, "Virtue and Identity," 71.

15. Keenan, "Proposing," 723–24. These four virtues and hope do not preclude love or charity, but allow love to be the basis of all virtues. Keenan writes: "Generally speaking, Roman Catholics tend to consider love as the basis of all virtues. For instance, Thomas distinguishes charity or Christian love from the four cardinal virtues. If we want to know what to do in the concrete, we must turn not to charity, which is about union with God, but to the cardinal virtues, which are about right living." 725.

16. William F. Lynch, *Images of Hope: Imagination as Healer of the Hopeless* (Baltimore: Helicon Press, 1965), 35. A fine analysis of Lynch's work is found in Gerald J. Bednar, *Faith As Imagination: The Contribution of William F. Lynch, S.J.* (Kansas City: Sheed and Ward, 1996).

17. I distinguish Christian hope here from existential or humanistic hope.

18. Lynch, *Images*, 23. Lynch powerfully explains that despair occurs because one imagines alone and cannot see outside the situation.

19. See Johann Metz, *Faith in History and Society: Toward a Practical Fundamental Theology*, trans. David Smith (New York: Seabury Press, 1980), 73; Ashley, *Interruptions*, 130.

20. Lynch, *Images*, 40.

21. Ibid., 40.

22. On hope and eschatology, see also Vincent J. Genovesi, SJ, *Expectant Creativity: The Action of Hope in Christian Ethics* (Lanham, MD: University Press of America, 1982).

23. For an overview of Aquinas's discussion of hope, see Romanus Cessario, "The Theological Virtue of Hope" (IIa IIai, qq.17–22), in *The Ethics of Aquinas*, ed. Stephen J. Pope (Washington, D.C.: Georgetown University Press, 2002), 232–43.

24. See Robert J. Schreiter, CPpS, *The Ministry of Reconciliation: Spirituality and Strategies* (Maryknoll, NY: Orbis Books, 1998), 70–82.

25. See also the passage in John 20: 24–29, in which Jesus invites Thomas to touch Jesus' hands and side.

26. Keenan, "Proposing," 724–25.

27. Ibid., 725.

28. Our love of God and God's love for us represents a prime relationship for Christians. We also live out this relationship with and through others. For Christians, charity is to be the foundation for all the virtues.

29. Margaret A. Farley, "Fragments for an Ethic of Commitment in Thomas

Aquinas," *Celebrating the Medieval Heritage*, ed. David Tracy. *Journal of Religion* (1978): S146–47.

30. Farley, "Fragments," S142.

31. See Margaret A. Farley, "How Shall We Love in a Postmodern World?" *The Annual of the Society of Christian Ethics* (Washinton, DC: Georgetown University Press, 1994): 3–19; Farley, "A Feminist Version of Respect for Persons," *Journal of Feminist Studies in Religion* 9 (Spring 1993): 182–98; Edith Wyschogrod, *Saints and Postmodernism* (Chicago: University of Chicago Press, 1990): 233–57. A history of the development of concern for the other in twentieth century philosophy can be found in Michael Theunissen, *The Other: Studies in the Social Ontology of Husserl, Heidegger, Sartre, and Buber*, trans. C. Macann (Cambridge: MIT Press, 1984).

32. We are here further enfleshing out the "embodied" relational agent discussed in chapter three.

33. We can, of course, use the other solely for our own needs. However, this would not then constitute fidelity or love.

34. For a discussion of sex and sexual intercourse, see, e.g., Vincent J. Genovesi, *In Pursuit of Love: Catholic Morality and Human Sexuality*, 2d ed. (Collegeville, MN: Liturgical Press, 1996); Fran Ferder and John Heagle, *Tender Fires: The Spiritual Promise of Sexuality* (New York: Crossroad Publ., 2002); Ronald Lawler, Joseph Boyle, Jr., and William E. May, *Catholic Sexual Ethics: A Summary, Explanation, & Defense,* 2d ed. (Huntington, IN: Our Sunday Visitor Publ., 1998); Christine Gudorf, *Body, Sex and Pleasure: Reconstructing Christian Sexual Ethics* (Cleveland: Pilgrim Press, 1994); James B. Nelson, *Embodiment: An Approach to Sexuality and Christian Theology* (Minneapolis: Augsburg Publ., 1978); James B. Nelson and Sandra P. Longfellow, ed. *Sexuality and the Sacred: Sources for Theological Reflection* (Louisville: Westminster/John Knox Press, 1994); Karen Lebacqz, "Appropriate Vulnerability: A Sexual Ethic for Singles," *The Christian Century* 104, no. 15 (6 May 1987): 435–438; and James F. Keenan, "The Open Debate: Moral Theology and the Lives of Gay and Lesbian Persons," *Theological Studies* 64 (2003): 127–50. For specific discussions about sexual expressions and HIV/AIDS, see, e.g., Kevin T. Kelly, *New Directions in Sexual Ethics: Moral Theology and the Challenge of AIDS* (London and Washington: Geoffrey Chapman, 1998); any of the excellent articles in James F. Keenan, ed., assisted by Jon D. Fuller, Lisa Sowle Cahill, and Kevin Kelly, *Catholic Ethicists on HIV/AIDS Prevention* (New York: Continuum, 2000), including Laurenti Magesa, "Recognizing the Reality of African Religion in Tanzania," 76–83; Eileen P. Flynn, "Teaching about HIV Prevention in an American Catholic College Classroom," 148–54; and Roger Burggraeve, "From Responsible to Meaningful Sexuality: An Ethics of Growth as an Ethics of Mercy for Young People in this Era of AIDS," 303–16. Official Church documents on sexuality include, among others, Paul VI, "Encyclical Letter on the Regulation of Births" (*Humanae Vitae*), 25 July 1968. English edition: *Vatican Council II: More Postconciliar Documents*, ed. Austin Flannery (Grand Rapids, MI: Eerdmans, 1982): 397–416; Congregation for the Doctrine of the Faith, "Declaration on Certain Questions Concerning Sexual Ethics" (*Persona humana*), 29 December 1975. English Edition: *Vatican Council II: More Postconciliar Documents*, ed. Austin Flannery (Grand Rapids, MI: Eerdmans, 1982): 77–96; and United States Catholic Council of Bishops (USCCB), *Human Sexuality: A Catholic Perspective for Education and Lifelong Learning*, 1997. Specific documents related to sexuality and HIV/AIDS in the U.S. include, among others, USCCB, *The Many Faces of AIDS: A Gospel Response*, A Statement

of the Administrative Board (Washington, D.C.: USCC, Inc., Nov. 1987); and National Conference Catholic Bishops (NCCB), *Called to Compassion and Responsibility: A Response to the HIV/AIDS Crisis* (Washington, D.C.: USCC, Inc., Nov. 1989).

35. This is not to suggest that even permanent committed relationships will not at some point need to be reassessed by the couple. We are constantly doing that in one way or another as we daily live out our commitments. But it is important to note that there may be times when a committed relationship changes to the point where the two are no longer able to live that commitment out. I will delve into this further in the discussion on the virtue of self-care, but I recognize its significance within any discussion of fidelity. Margaret Farley discusses the nuances of fidelity and how commitments evolve and change in *Personal Commitments*.

36. Hope and imagination are crucial here, and we will discuss imagination further within our exploration of the virtue of prudence.

37. Keenan, "Proposing," 727.

38. See Margaret A. Farley, "Feminism and Universal Morality," in *Prospects for a Common Morality*, ed. G. Outka and J. Reeder (Princeton: Princeton University Press, 1993): 170–90; Farley, "A Feminist Version of Respect for Persons," *Journal of Feminist Studies in Religion* 9 (Spring/Fall, 1993): 182–98; Barbara Hilkert Andolsen, "Agape in Feminist Ethics," *Journal of Religious Ethics* 9.1 (Spring 1981): 69–83.

39. See David Hollenbach, *The Common Good and Christian Ethics* (New York: Cambridge University Press, 2002); Hollenbach, *The Common Good in a Divided Society* (Santa Clara, CA: Santa Clara University, 1999); Robert F. Drinan, *The Mobilization of Shame: A World View of Human Rights* (New Haven, Conn: Yale University Press, 2001); Martha C. Nussbaum, *Sex and Social Justice* (New York: Oxford University Press, 1999); and Nussbaum, *Women and Human Development: The Capabilities Approach* (Cambridge, New York: Cambridge University Press, 2000).

40. Edward Collins Vacek, SJ, *Love, Human and Divine: The Heart of Christian Ethics* (Washington, DC: Georgetown University Press, 1994).

41. Ibid., 262–263. Self-care is a term that is also used in professional ethics. See Katherine M. Clarke, "Lessons from Feminist Therapy for Ministerial Ethics," *Journal of Pastoral Care* 48 (1994): 233–42.

42. See Keenan, "Proposing," 726–28. Keenan's remarks about Aquinas and self-care are helpful: "The concern for self-care runs throughout the *Summa*, from 1.5.1 corp and 48.1, which describe how all nature seeks its own perfection, to 1-2.27.3 that insists it is natural to prefer oneself over others, and 29.4 that states the impossibility of hating oneself. In 2-2, Aquinas argues that though inordinate self-love is the source of sin (25.4, 28.4 ad 1), self-love belongs to the order of charity and is prior to neighbor love (25.12, 26.4). He adds that charity is the source of peace which aims at ending conflict not only with others but also within oneself (29.1). By introducing self-care into the constellation of the cardinal virtues I believe I am developing Thomas's own thoughts." See also Aquinas' argument against suicide in terms of both justice (depriving the common good) and self-care (doing harm to oneself). *ST* 2–2.64.5 ad 1. See also Stephen Pope, *The Evolution of Altruism and the Ordering of Love* (Washington, DC: Georgetown University Press, 1994); and Pope, "Expressive Individualism and True Self-Love: A Thomistic Perspective," *Journal of Religion* 71.3 (1991): 384–99.

43. Roger Burggraeve, "From Responsible to Meaningful Sexuality: An Ethics of Growth as an Ethics of Mercy for Young People in this Era of AIDS," in *Catholic Ethicists on HIV/AIDS Prevention*, ed. James F. Keenan et al., 308.

44. Ibid., 303–16; see also "Une Ethique de miséricorde," *Lumen Vitae: Revue internationale de catéchèse et de pastorale* 49 (September 1994): 281–96; and "Prohibitions and Taste: Bipolarity in Christian Ethics," *Ethical Perspectives* 1 (September 1994): 130–44.

45. Burggraeve, "From Responsible to Meaningful Sexuality," 304, 306. In "negative" terms, these may be called the "do no-harm" and "no-violence" principles. Neither person is to harm himself or to harm the other and neither person may be coerced or demeaned. Pope Pope Paul VI's "Encyclical Letter on the Regulation of Births," *Humanae Vitae*, 25 July 1968, English ed., *Vatican Council II: More Postconciliar Documents*, ed. Austin Flannery (Grand Rapids, MI: Eerdmans Publ., 1982): 397–416, explicitly prohibits artificial means that would prevent new life in any act of sexual intercourse. This is to protect the unitive and procreative elements of a marriage act. However, the reality is that many acts of intercourse take place outside of permanent commitments. I am not promoting sex outside of permanent commitment, but rather acknowledging a reality in our world today. I am simply describing one means toward protecting persons from HIV and certain death. This is an ongoing conversation among many theologians (for example, James Keenan, Kevin Kelly, and Roger Burggraeve) as well as Catholic health care professionals (for example, Jon Fuller, MD, Paul Farmer, MD). Articles that engage the question of condoms and church teaching and responses in this age of AIDS include, but are not limited to, Jon Fuller and James Keenan, "Church Politics and HIV Prevention: Why Is the Condom Question So Significant and So Neuralgic?"; Fuller and Keenan, "Condoms, Catholics and HIV/AIDS Prevention," *The Furrow* 52:9 (Sept. 2001): 459–67; Kevin T. Kelly, *New Directions in Sexual Ethics*, 196–206; James Keenan, "Prophylactics, Toleration, and Cooperation: Contemporary Problems and Traditional Principles," *International Philosophical Quarterly* 28 (1988): 201–20; Enda McDonagh, "Theology in a Time of AIDS," *Irish Theological Quarterly* 60 (1994): 81–99; Hans Rotter, "AIDS: Some Theological and Pastoral Considerations," *Theology Digest* 39 (1992): 235–39; Bishop Anthony M. Pilla, "Statement on Developing an Approach by the Church to AIDS Education," *Origins* 16 (1987): 692–93; James Drane, "Condoms, AIDS, and Catholic Ethics," *Commonweal* 189 (1991): 188–92.

46. Burggraeve, "From Responsible to Meaningful Sexuality," 307.

47. Keenan, "Proposing," 724. See also Keenan, "Virtue and Identity," 74–75.

48. Aquinas, IIa IIae, q. 58, a. 1. Aquinas' definition follows Justinian's *Digest*. See Jean Porter, "The Virtue of Justice (IIa IIae, qq. 58–122)," in *The Ethics of Aquinas*, ed. Stephen J. Pope (Washington, D.C.: Georgetown University Press, 2002), 273. In her essay, Porter offers an extensive treatment of the complexity of Aquinas' work on justice.

49. For example, defending someone wrongly accused of a crime is a requirement of justice and of charity. However, staying at the bedside of a person suffering from cancer is a call of charity but not necessarily a call of justice.

50. Karen Lebacqz, "Justice," in *Christian Ethics: An Introduction*, ed. Bernard Hoose (Collegeville, MN: The Liturgical Press, 1998), 169. Michael H. Crosby, OFM, Cap. also reminds us that "the two main Hebrew words for 'justice,' *sedeq* and *sedaqa*, refer to the many-faceted dimensions of both divine and human justice as well

as to the works of justice (Exod 9:27; Prov 10: 25; Ps 18:21–25). Both words, despite their nuances, articulate various demands related to *relationships*. The experiential and expressive dimensions of a justice spirituality probably are best revealed in the prophetic injunction: To know Yahweh is to do justice (see Jer 22:13–16). To be in relationship with God demands the expression of this experience in the promotion of relationships of interhuman justice." "Justice," *The New Dictionary of Catholic Spirituality* ed. Michael Downey (Collegeville, MN: Liturgical Press, 1993), 581.

51. Jeffrey Weeks, *Invented Moralities: Sexual Values in an Age of Uncertainty* (New York: Columbia University Press, 1995), 72.

52. Farley, "New Patterns of Relationship: Beginnings of a Moral Revolution," *Theological Studies* 36 (1975): 646.

53. Crosby, "Justice," 579.

54. NCCB, *Economic Justice for All: Pastoral Letter on Catholic Social Teaching and the U.S. Economy* (Washington, DC: USCC, 1986), 24.

55. Cahill, "AIDS, Justice, and the Common Good," *Catholic Ethicists*, 287–88.

56. Synod of Bishops, introduction to *Justice in the World 1971*, in *Catholic Social Thought: The Documentary Heritage*, ed. David J. O'Brien and Thomas A. Shannon (Maryknoll, NY: Orbis Books, 1992).

57. Lebacqz, "Justice," 168.

58. Excellent presentations on the Trinity have emerged in recent years, most notably from Catherine Mowry LaCugna, *God for Us: The Trinity and Christian Life* (San Francisco: Harper, 1991) and Elizabeth A. Johnson, *She Who Is: The Mystery of God in a Feminist Theological Perspective* (New York: Crossroad, 1992).

59. Synod of Bishops, introduction to *Justice in the World 1971*.

60. I will develop this topic in the final chapter.

61. The popular media has an agenda, as do most media. Knowing the ideological, religious and other angles from which information systems operate is part of critical analysis.

62. This is not to say that HIV/AIDS only occurs outside of comfortable places. Persons living with AIDS can live in suburbs and rural areas as well as in urban or developing areas. The point is simply that many persons with HIV/AIDS are on the margins of society.

63. Solidarity also has a more active dimension. We will discuss solidarity further in chapter 6.

64. Bernard Williams writes that the claim of equality emerges from within as justice orders the interior dispositions of the person: "Justice as a Virtue," in *Essays on Aristotle's Ethics*, ed. Amélie Oksenberg Rorty (Berkeley: University of California, 1980), 189–99.

65. Crosby, "Justice," 582.

66. An indirect benefit of a spirit of interiority is that it can support proper self-care. To the extent that it can help to prevent burnout, self-care is also an element of justice.

67. The common good, allowing for the full human flourishing of each and all, is a principle of Catholic social teaching. It is particularly exhorted in regard to the economic sphere in NCCB, *Economic Justice for All*.

68. Tina Rosenberg, "Look at Brazil," *The New York Times Magazine*, 28 January 2001, 26.

69. This is helping some countries. However, many countries still cannot afford the drugs on their own. A global effort is required to make it possible for more per-

sons to access the drugs. For information on pharmaceuticals and AIDS drug price cuts, see, for example, John Donnelly, "Deal on AIDS Drugs Fuels Push for More Funds: Indian Firm Agrees to Provide Treatment Cheaply to Charity," *Boston Globe* 8 February 2001. This is the story of the Bombay-based Cipla company which has lowered the cost of drug treatment; Reuters, "Merck Leads New Round of AIDS Drug Price Cuts," March 7, 2001; Helene Cooper, Rachel Zimmerman and Laurie McGinley, "AIDS Epidemic Puts Drug Firms in a Vise: Treatment vs. Profits," *Wall Street Journal*, 2 March 2001; available at http://interactive.wsj.com/articles/ SB983487988418159849.htm.; Internet; accessed 2 March 2001; and Mark Schoofs and Michael Waldholz, "Price War Breaks Out Over AIDS Drugs in Africa as Generics Present Challenge," *Wall Street Journal*, 7 March 2001.

70. Keenan, "Proposing Cardinal Virtues," 725. Spohn offers a similar insight in "The Return of Virtue Ethics," 72.

71. Aquinas, Ia IIae, q.57, a.4. Aquinas is here invoking Aristotle's claim (*Metaph.* 9.8 1050a30-b2). See also Keenan, "The Virtue of Prudence (IIa IIae, qq.47–56)," in *The Ethics of Aquinas*, ed. Stephen J. Pope (Washington, DC: Georgetown University Press, 2002), 259.

72. Aquinas, Ia IIae, q.57, a.4 ad 3 cited in Keenan, "The Virtue of Prudence," 259. Keenan also sums up well that prudence "guides the agent to living a self-directed life that seeks integration."

73. Yves R. Simon, *The Definition of Moral Virtue*, ed. Vukan Kuic (New York: Fordham University Press, 1986), 96–98.

74. Keenan, "Virtue of Prudence," 259. See also Daniel Mark Nelson, *The Priority of Prudence* (University Park: Pennsylvania State University Press, 1992).

75. Contemporary writing on this topic has included Mary Jo Iozzio, *Self-Determination and the Moral Act: A Study of the Contributions of Odon Lottin (OSB)* (Leuven: Peeters, 1995) and Klaus Demmer, "La competenza normativa del magistero ecclesiastico in morale," *Fede cristiana e agire morale*, ed. Klaus Demmer and Bruno Schuller (Assisi: Cittadella Editrice, 1980),144–71. There has also been more writing recently on the relationship between prudence and natural law and the virtues. See Dennis Billy, "Aquinas on the Relations of Prudence," *Studia Moralia* 33 (1995): 250; and Maria Carl, "Law, Virtue, and Happiness in Aquinas' Moral Theory," *Thomist* 61 (1997): 427.

76. Aquinas, *ST* IIa IIae, q.47, a.7.

77. Keenan, "Virtue of Prudence," 266, Aquinas, Ia IIae, q.65, a.2: "Now for prudence to proceed aright, it is much more necessary that man be well disposed toward his ultimate end, which is the effect of charity, than that he be well disposed in respect of other ends, which is the effect of moral virtue."

78. This determination can be for a given situation.

79. Yves R. Simon, *The Definition of Moral Virtue*, 129.

80. This may be, in part, because some consider that to be prudent is to follow some pre-determined lines of acceptability. I instead want to also emphasize that prudence offers much creative possibility.

81. I add the term "moral" to imagination to further focus our attention on the way we live our life as Christians.

82. In this section I use the terms imagination, moral imagination and Christian imagination interchangeably.

83. Philip S. Keane, SS., *Christian Ethics and Imagination: A Theological Inquiry* (New York: Paulist Press, 1984), 81.

84. William Spohn uses this term and description in *Go and Do Likewise*, 56, when commenting on William F. Lynch's work on the imagination, *Images of Hope: Imagination as Healer of the Hopeless* (Notre Dame: University of Notre Dame Press, 1974).

85. Lynch, *Images of Hope*, 35.

86. A key text on the analogical imagination is David Tracy, *The Analogical Imagination: Christian Theology and the Culture of Pluralism* (New York: Crossroad, 1981). See also Spohn, *Go and Do Likewise*.

87. Spohn, *Go and Do Likewise*, 4.

88. Moser and Leers, *Moral Theology: Dead Ends and Alternatives*, 166–67.

5. Discipleship

1. For helpful historical explanations of the separation of moral theology and spirituality and of efforts to reintegrate them, see James F. Keenan, SJ, "Spirituality and Morality: What's the Difference?" in *Method and Catholic Moral Theology: The Ongoing Reconstruction*, ed. Todd A. Salzman (Omaha, NE: Creighton University Press, 1999), 87–102, and "Ethics and Spirituality: Historical Distinctions and Contemporary Challenges," *Listening* (Fall 1999): 167–79; and Jean Porter, "Virtue Ethics and Its Significance for Spirituality," *The Way* 88, Suppl. (Spring 1997): 26–35. Other recent contributions have included Edward C. Vacek, *Love, Human and Divine: The Heart of Christian Ethics* (Washington, DC: Georgetown University Press, 1994); Mark O'Keefe, OSB, *Becoming Good, Becoming Holy: On the Relationship of Christian Ethics and Spirituality* (New York: Paulist Press, 1995); Ronald Rolheiser, *The Holy Longing: The Search for a Christian Spirituality* (New York: Doubleday, 1999); other essays in *Method and Catholic Moral Theology: The Ongoing Reconstruction*; and essays in *Spirituality and Moral Theology: Essays from a Pastoral Perspective*, ed. James Keating (New York: Paulist Press, 2000).

2. Keenan, "Spirituality and Morality," 97. See also Fritz Tillmann, *The Master Calls: A Handbook of Christian Living* (Baltimore: Helicon Press, 1960).

3. Bernard Häring, *The Law of Christ* (Westminster, MD: Newman Press, 1961).

4. See William C. Spohn, *Go and Do Likewise: Jesus and Ethics* (New York: Continuum, 2000); Richard M Gula, *The Call to Holiness: Embracing a Fully Christian Life* (New York: Paulist Press, 2003); and Timothy E. O'Connell, *Making Disciples: A Handbook of Christian Moral Formation* (New York: Crossroad Publishing, 1998).

5. I am referring here to the lived experience of spirituality. Gula writes that spirituality "expresses a way of life animated by the longings of a restless human spirit. Or, to be more formal about it, spirituality designates a way of living that strives to integrate our diverse experiences into a meaningful whole by connecting all of life to what we believe gives ultimate meaning and value to our lives." *The Call to Holiness*, 18. Gula's definition is influenced by the work of Sandra Schneiders. See especially "Theology and Spirituality: Strangers, Rivals, or Partners?" *Horizons* 13 (Fall 1986): 266, and "Spirituality in the Academy," *Theological Studies* 50, no. 4 (1989): 676–97, at 684. For resources on the academic discipline of spirituality one can begin with two essays by Sandra Schneiders, "Spirituality in the Academy," 676–97, and "Spirituality as an Academic Discipline: Reflections from Experience," in *Broken and Whole: Essays on Religion and the Body*, ed. Maureen A. Tilley and Susan A. Ross (Lanham, MD: University Press of America, 1993), 207–18.

6. David Lonsdale, *Eyes to See, Ears to Hear* (Chicago: Loyola University Press, 1990), 1–3.

7. Philip Sheldrake, *Spirituality and Theology: Christian Living and the Doctrine of God* (Maryknoll, NY: Orbis Books, 1998), 34–35.

8. Gula, *The Call to Holiness*, 21. It is important to note that Gula's definition also describes the moral life.

9. Mark O'Keefe, "Liturgical Preaching and the Moral Life of Christians," in *Spirituality and Moral Theology: Essays from a Pastoral Perspective*, 44.

10. Gula, *The Call to Holiness*, 37–38.

11. This is certainly not an exhaustive account. Rather, it is an opening discussion on six essential elements for this age of AIDS.

12. The initiative for discipleship comes from Jesus. The disciples did not choose the master first; they were chosen. This is different from discipleship in Rabbinic Judaism. See Thomas P. Rausch, "Discipleship," in *The New Dictionary of Catholic Spirituality*, ed. Michael Downey (Collegeville, MN: Liturgical Press, 1993), 281.

13. This is the Christian vocation—to make God's love present to people.

14. This is, of course, a process. God is continually reaching out to us in love, and we are at varying levels of accepting and responding to that love. This is a life-long journey for the Christian.

15. Here we find a connection again to the life of virtue, where we relate generally, particularly, and uniquely to others, to God, and to ourselves.

16. It must also be noted here that there are a variety of spiritualities even within Christian spirituality. A Christian spirituality may be, among other things, Franciscan, Benedictine, lay, marital, feminist, Latino, or African. This diversity reminds us that we meet and respond to God and neighbor in different contexts. For example, while encompassing all of the above aspects of discipleship, a Franciscan spirituality would have a flavor different from that of a Benedictine spirituality. The difference comes in the way the founders of the Franciscans and Benedictines heard the Spirit calling them forth to love in the world around them. For each of us today, experiences, disposition, and specific dimensions of our worship may cause us to lean more toward one particular spirituality than another.

17. We must be mindful, too, that faith is also a growth process. At various points in our lives we may be more connected to certain persons and dimensions of the Trinity than to others. Thus a person is not denying the Spirit if her personal prayer is directed to Jesus Christ rather than to the Spirit, and vice versa.

18. Vincent Macnamara, "The Moral Journey," *The Way* 88, Suppl. (Spring 1997): 9.

19. See Sandra M. Schneiders, *The Revelatory Text: Interpreting the New Testament as Sacred Scripture*, 2nd ed. (Collegeville, MN: Liturgical Press, 1999).

20. Spohn, *Go and Do Likewise*, 10–11.

21. Spohn speaks to this topic in detail. *Go and Do Likewise*, 10.

22. Even if persons have experienced considerable suffering, it is experiences of love that may hold out a possibility and desire for a changed situation, for a different way to live. This is, of course, dependent on many factors, including a person's temperament and current situation. Nevertheless, the experience of love is a powerful factor, perhaps the most powerful factor, along with hope, for resisting suffering. However, as I will attend to later, for a variety of reasons we do not really engage the world's suffering and thus do not bring that love to bear upon pain or injustices.

23. For a discussion of discernment and conscience formation, see Richard M.

Gula, *Moral Discernment* (New York: Paulist Press, 1997); *The Call to Holiness*, 201–11; and Charles E. Curran, *The Catholic Moral Tradition Today: A Synthesis* (Washington, DC: Georgetown University Press, 1999), 182–90.

24. Anne E. Patrick, "Ethics and Spirituality: The Social Justice Connection," *The Way* 63, Suppl. (1988): 113–14.

25. Rebecca S. Chopp, "Praxis," in *The New Dictionary of Catholic Spirituality*, ed. Michael Downey (Collegeville, MN: Liturgical Press, 1993), 756.

26. Ibid., 756.

27. Ibid., 764.

28. Ibid., 756.

29. Patrick, "Ethics and Spirituality," 113–14.

30. Macnamara, "The Moral Journey," 7.

31. Macnamara writes: "It is a task—and not just an intellectual task—to discover and acknowledge in our hearts the truth for our individual lives. Moral truth is difficult to allow in because it commits us and we may not be able to bear the reality. We are entangled in many biases that distort judgment—the biases of nation, tribe, group, gender, profession, personal taste. We are more easily beguiled by the sirens of our surface desires than by the gentle call within us to truth and goodness. We are invested emotionally in what feeds our ego and will deny the claims of whatever threatens it" ("The Moral Journey," 9–10). In addition to these biases, we must acknowledge the reality of sin and of our failure at times to bother to love. Included at the systemic or personal level of sin is any deliberate exclusion, marginalization, or stigmatization for the purpose of domination.

32. See Dietrich Bonhoeffer, *The Cost of Discipleship* (New York: Macmillan, 1959).

6. Memory, Narrative, and Solidarity

1. Metz examines the most fundamental features of the human being through the lens of memory, narrative, and solidarity. These categories are not meant to be exhaustive, but are a means of probing one's relationship to God and to one another. The terms are not linear, but form a spiral, each illuminating a way to deeper being and fuller action. The categories of memory, narrative, and solidarity offer an imaginative way to probe discipleship, opening up traditional resources and inviting innovative possibilities, offering both resources and guides for living and ministering in our world today. Metz writes about these categories, especially in the last section of *Faith in History and Society: Toward a Practical Fundamental Theology*, trans. David Smith (New York: Seabury Press), 1980. The discussion can be found under the heading of "categories." J. Matthew Ashley discusses these categories in *Interruptions: Mysticism, Politics, and Theology in the Work of Johann Baptist Metz* (Notre Dame, IN: University of Notre Dame Press, 1998). While beginning with Metz's insights, I will include within these categories insights from various other writers.

2. Paul J. Philibert, OP, writes that "Memory is the ability to recall images of events and to recognize them as having happened in the past. Like imagination, memory is linked to the translation of physical objects into the state of mental images and ideas. Memory is marked, however, by the precise awareness that its images are objects that were presented in the past. . . . Memory is a psychosomatic phenomenon, having features that are both mental and bodily. Psychically, memory

involves four steps: (a) learning through impressions that fix an experience in consciousness; (b) retention by marking particular images as needed for future use; (c) restoration of past images within the field of awareness; (d) attributing to images the quality of belonging to the past by putting them in their historical setting." "Memory," *The New Dictionary of Catholic Spirituality*, ed. Michael Downey (Collegeville, MN: Liturgical Press, 1993), 651–52.

3. Ashley, *Interruptions*, 35.

4. Johann Baptist Metz, *A Passion for God: The Mystical-Political Dimension of Christianity*, trans J. Matthew Ashley (New York: Paulist Press, 1998), 2. Metz further writes, "This biographical background shines through all my theological work, even to this day. In it, for example, the category of memory plays a central role; my work does not want to let go of the apocalyptic metaphors of the history of faith, and it mistrusts an idealistically smoothed out eschatology. . . . Whoever talks about God in Jesus' sense will always take into account the way one's own pre-formulated certainties are wounded by the misfortune of others" (2).

5. Ashley, commenting on Metz, writes: "For Christians the paradigmatic memory is the *memoria passionis et resurrectionis Jesu Christi*, a memory which as we narrate and commemorate it sacramentally, continually opens us up to other crucified persons" (*Interruptions*, 161).

6. Jean-Marc Ela, "Christianity and Liberation in Africa," in *Paths of African Theology*, ed. Rosino Gibellini (Maryknoll, NY: Orbis Books, 1994), 146.

7. Mercy Amba Oduyoye, "Feminist Theology in an African Perspective" in *Paths of African Theology*, ed. Rosino Gibellini (Maryknoll, NY: Orbis Books, 1994), 178. The context for her remarks is gender issues related to alienation and oppression.

8. In this discussion of memory, it is important to remember that for some, memories of pain and suffering are destructive if they are not held gently and if the person is not helped to describe the memory in a safe and welcoming space. Dangerous memories of suffering require healing, and this too takes time. Yet if we do not acknowledge the dangerous memories of our past and present history, we will also not respond to them.

9. Belden C. Lane, "Narrative," in *The New Dictionary of Catholic Spirituality*, ed. Michael Downey (Collegeville, MN: Liturgical Press, 1993), 696.

10. A community sharing of faith stories also has great ecumenical potential.

11. Robert J. Schreiter, CPPS, *The Ministry of Reconciliation: Spirituality and Strategies* (Maryknoll, NY: Orbis Books, 2000), 19–20.

12. Johann Baptist Metz, "God and the Evil of This World, Forgotten, Unforgettable Theodicy," in *The Return of the Plague*, ed. Jose Oscar Beozzo and Virgil Elizondo (London: SCM Press, 1997), 6. A narrative that illustrates this gaze of love is the parable of the Good Samaritan. Metz writes that here we have "one who is disregarded by the priest and the levite 'in the interest of higher things.' Those who look for 'God' as Jesus understands God do not know 'any higher interest' to excuse them here. This authority of the sufferer is the only authority in which the authority of the God who judges manifests itself in the world for all human beings (Matt. 25:31–46). Conscience constitutes itself in obedience to it, and what we call its voice is our reaction to a visitation by this suffering of others" (6). This is a "dangerous narrative," for it reminds us that no institutional practice is greater than the people of God. It reminds us how concretely our love of neighbor is our love of God.

13. Removing borders here is not to prevent identity but to encourage openness. The balance needs to be maintained.

14. Christine D. Pohl, *Making Room: Recovering Hospitality as a Christian Tradition* (Grand Rapids, MI: Eerdmans, 1999), 174.

15. For further exploration of the virtue of mercy, see Daniel J. Harrington, SJ, and James F. Keenan, SJ, *Jesus and Virtue Ethics: Building Bridges Between New Testament Studies and Moral Theology* (Lanham, MD: Sheed & Ward, 2002).

16. Mary Catherine Hilkert, *Naming Grace: Preaching and the Sacramental Imagination* (New York: Continuum, 1997).

17. Lane, "Narrative," 696.

18. Hilkert, *Naming Grace*, 126.

19. This is much like our example in Chapter 2 of slave narratives passed down from one generation to the next.

20. As quoted in Raymond Flynn and Robin Moore, *The Accidental Pope* (New York: St. Martin's Press, 2000).

21. Roberto S. Goizueta, "Solidarity," in *The New Dictionary of Catholic Spirituality*, ed. Michael Downey (Collegeville, MN: Liturgical Press, 1993), 906.

22. William C. Spohn, *Go and Do Likewise: Jesus and Ethics* (New York: Continuum, 2000), 180.

23. For a fine exposition of the Trinity, mutuality, and communion, see Catherine Mowry LaCugna, *God for Us: The Trinity and Christian Life* (San Francisco: Harper, 1991).

24. Goizueta, "Solidarity," in *The New Dictionary of Catholic Spirituality*, ed. Michael Downey (Collegeville, MN: Liturgical Press, 1993), 906.

25. Simone Weil, *Waiting for God*, trans. Emma Craufurd (New York: Harper & Row, 1973), 115. Weil fills out this question in her essay. She writes:

> In the first legend of the Grail it is said that the Grail (the miraculous vessel that satisfies all hunger by virtue of the consecrated Host) belongs to the first comer who asks the guardian of the vessel, a king three-quarters paralyzed by the most painful wound, "What are you going through?" The love of neighbor in all its fullness simply means being able to say to him: "What are you going through?" It is a recognition that the sufferer exists, not only as a unit in a collection, or a specimen from the social category labeled "unfortunate," but as a man, exactly like us, who was one day stamped with a special mark by affliction. For this reason it is enough, but it is indispensable, to know how to look at him in a certain way. The way of looking is first of all attentive. The soul empties itself of its own contents in order to receive into itself the being it is looking at, just as he is, in all his truth. Only he who is capable of attention can do this.

26. Johann Baptist Metz, "Communicating a Dangerous Memory," in *Communicating a Dangerous Memory: Soundings in Political Theology*, ed. Fred Lawrence (Atlanta: Scholars Press, 1987), 40.

27. John Paul II, *Sollicitudo Rei Socialis*, in *Catholic Social Thought: The Documentary Heritage*, eds. David J. O'Brien and Thomas A. Shannon (Maryknoll, NY: Orbis Books, 1992), no. 39. Other Church documents related to solidarity include, among others, Second Vatican Council, *Gaudium et Spes*, Pope Paul VI, *Populorum Progressio*; and Pope John Paul II, *Laborem Exercens*, in *Catholic Social Thought: The Documentary Heritage*.

28. Jon Sobrino, "Bearing with One Another in Faith," in *Theology of Christian*

Solidarity, ed. Jon Sobrino and Juan Hernández Pico, trans. Phillip Berryman (Mary-knoll, NY: Orbis Books, 1985), 11.

29. Ibid., 10–11.

30. Ibid., 11.

31. Anne E. Patrick, *Liberating Conscience: Feminist Explorations in Catholic Moral Theology* (New York: Continuum, 1997), 195.

32. Goizueta, "Solidarity," 906.

33. Patrick, *Liberating Conscience*, 195.

34. John Paul II, *Sollicitudo Rei Socialis*, in *Catholic Social Thought: The Documentary Heritage*, no. 39.

35. Ada María Isasi-Díaz, "Solidarity: Love of Neighbor in the 1980s," in *Lift Every Voice: Constructing Christian Theologies from the Underside*, ed. Susan Brooks Thistlethwaite and Mary Potter Engel (San Francisco: Harper & Row, 1990), 35.

36. Some may die, in the many ways people die—physically, emotionally, psychologically, relationally.

37. Schreiter, *The Ministry of Reconciliation*, 20.

7. Bearing Witness

1. I will be summarizing Kaleeba's story from a number of sources. They include Noerine Kaleeba, *We Miss You All* (Harare, Zimbabwe: Women and AIDS Support Network, 1991); Noerine Kaleeba, Sunanda Ray, and Brigid Willmore, *We Miss You All: AIDS in the Family* (Kampala: Marianum Press, 1993); M. H. Merson, *TASO Uganda: The Inside Story* (Kampala: Marianum Press, 1995); Kevin T. Kelly, *New Directions in Sexual Ethics: Moral Theology and the Challenge of AIDS* (London and Washington: Geoffrey Chapman, 1998), 188–92; John Mary Waliggo, "A Woman Confronts Social Stigma in Uganda," in *Catholic Ethicists on HIV/AIDS Prevention*, ed. James F. Keenan, assisted by Jon D. Fuller, Lisa Sowle Cahill, and Kevin Kelly (New York: Continuum, 2000), 48–56.

2. Waliggo, "A Woman Confronts Social Stigma in Uganda," 49.

3. Noerine Kaleeba, Address to the World Health Assembly, May 2001; available at http://www.unaids.org/whatsnew/speeches/eng/kaleeba1405who.htm; Internet; accessed July 2003.

4. Kelly, *New Directions in Sexual Ethics*, 189.

5. Ibid., 189. Kelly adds that "Ironically, it was only much later that Noerine discovered that Chris had probably been infected with HIV due to a blood transfusion (8 units) he had received from his brother after he had been knocked down by a bus in 1983. That brother died of AIDS the year after Chris." 189.

6. Ibid., 190.

7. Kaleeba, Address to World Health Assembly, May 2001.

8. Waliggo, "A Woman Confronts Social Stigma in Uganda," 50.

9. Ibid., 51. The categories are further explained on 51–55.

10. Kaleeba, "Stigma and AIDS," keynote address; available at http://www.hdnet.org/Stigma/Meeting%20Agenda%20and%20presentations/Keynote%20address.html; Internet; accessed July 2003.

11. Kelly, *New Directions in Sexual Ethics*, 191. In *We Miss You All*, Noerine writes that "The public health messages were saying 'Beware of AIDS. AIDS kills.' 'You catch it and you are as good as dead.' There were no messages for those peo-

ple who were already infected. What was implied was that people who were already infected should die and get it over. People with HIV and AIDS were seen as dying. We adopted the slogan of 'Living positively with AIDS' in direct defiance of that perception. We emphasized *living* rather than *dying* with AIDS. For us it was the quality rather than the quantity of life which was important." 79–80.

12. Waliggo, "A Woman Confronts Social Stigma in Uganda," 53.

13. Kaleeba, *We Miss You All*, 79–80.

14. See, for example, Noerine Kaleeba, Joyce Namulondo Kadowe, Daniel Kalinaki, and Glen Williams, *Open Secret: People Facing Up to HIV and AIDS in Uganda*, Strategies for Hope Series, no. 15 (London: ACTIONAID, 2000). The book provides a helpful overview of the situation of AIDS in Uganda and the various initiatives set in place to positively confront AIDS. See 21–23 for specific information on TASO.

15. Kaleeba, Address to World Health Assembly, May 2001.

16. Noerine Kaleeba, quoted in "Profile: International Dream Team: She's the One," in *Pox: Health, Hope and HIV* (July 1998); available at http://www.poxy.com; Internet; accessed 19 June 2003.

17. Kaleeba, Address to World Health Assembly, May 2001.

18. Kaleeba, Address to World Health Assembly, May 2001. She states further: "For example, if we kept parents alive even for five extra years we would have less to worry about orphans because children would grow up with parental guidance and love. Second, intensify global efforts to find a vaccine. Invest more in the science but also increase developing country involvement. Most importantly involve the community more; they may not know the science but they hold the key to a successful vaccine program. Address some of the most outstanding issues which might hinder community involvement, particularly issues around care and support for vaccine participants."

19. Kaleeba's story is remarkably different from the cases presented in Linda Hogan, "An Irish Nun Living with Contradictions: Responding to HIV/AIDS in the Context of Church Teaching," in *Catholic Ethicists on HIV/AIDS Prevention*, 41–47, and Nicholas Peter Harvey, "Listening in England to a Woman's Life Experience," in *Catholic Ethicists on HIV/AIDS Prevention*, 70–75. In both of these cases the women had no experiences of solidarity. The nun is marginalized by a community that is marginalized by its bishop. The woman in Harvey's story is still challenged by a memory that without solidarity crushes and shatters.

20. Waliggo, "A Woman Confronts Social Stigma in Uganda," 51.

21. Tracy Kidder, "The Good Doctor," *New Yorker*, 10 July 2000, 57. Tracy Kidder followed this article with a book on Paul Farmer. See also Tracy Kidder, *Mountains Beyond Mountains: The Quest of Dr. Paul Farmer, A Man Who Would Cure the World* (New York: Random House: 2003).

22. Kidder, "The Good Doctor," 57.

23. Ibid.

24. Ibid.

25. Ibid., 42.

26. The roots of Partners in Health are further described in a brochure published by the organization:

Though founded in 1987, Partners in Health's roots go back to 1983 when we began working with a group of community activists based in the central plateau of Haiti. Members of the collective that is now called "Zanmi Lasante" . . .

had been working in the region since 1956 when Haiti's largest river was dammed as part of an international development project. Like many other large and poorly planned foreign aid projects, this one harmed the local communities. The village of Cange, for example, was flooded, leaving its inhabitants—all of whom were peasant farmers—landless. The people were not reimbursed for their losses, and the electricity generated by the hydroelectric dam was consumed, far away, in the capital city. For years Cange consisted of a few shanties and a dispirited core of "water refugees" who had been forced to move to less fertile land as a result of the dam. But with the financial and moral support of many Haitians and North Americans, Zanmi Lasante and the people of Cange built a large school and completed a water project to bring clean water to the dusty settlement. Cange began to resemble a real village. Partners in Health grew out of this work and determination.

27. Brochure, Partners in Health. These have culminated in a Health Surveillance Project, the Bon Sauveur Health Clinic, a clinical laboratory, a water sanitation project, education projects, and a TB project.

28. Brochure, Partners in Health.

29. Ibid.

30. Paul Farmer, "Medicine and Social Justice," *America*, 15 July 1995, 14. Farmer writes: "Over the past decade, Partners in Health has joined local community health activists to provide basic primary care and preventive services to poor communities in Mexico, Peru and especially Haiti—offering what we have termed pragmatic solidarity. As often as not, our medical efforts have been informed by certain insights from liberation theology."

31. Ibid., 13–17. The specific question he asks is, "How would a health intervention inspired by liberation theology be different from those with more conventional underpinnings?"(14).

32. Ibid., 13–14.

33. See Kidder, "The Good Doctor," 42. Treatable conditions include malaria and tuberculosis. Farmer also considers HIV+ to be a treatable condition.

34. Cited in Farmer, "Medicine and Social Justice," 13.

35. Ibid., 17.

36. Ibid.

37. Paul Farmer, "Prevention Without Treatment Is Not Sustainable," *National AIDS Bulletin* (Australia) 13, no. 6 (2000): 6, 7. This paper was presented at the XIII International AIDS Conference in Durban, South Africa. A lengthier piece that includes this information is found in Paul Farmer, "Preface to the Paperback Edition," in *Infections and Inequalities: The Modern Plagues* (Berkeley, CA: University of California Press, 1999), xx–xxviii.

38. Farmer, "Preface to the Paperback Edition," *Infections and Inequalities*, xxv–xxvi. The term "cultural beliefs" in this citation includes a footnote referring the reader to a review of data supporting this claim. This review can be found in Paul Farmer, M. Connors, and J. Simmons, eds., *Women, Poverty, and AIDS: Sex, Drugs, and Structural Violence* (Monroe, ME: Common Courage Press, 1996).

39. Farmer, *Infections and Inequalities*, xxvii.

40. Ibid., xxvi.

41. Paul Farmer, "Revealing and Critiquing Inequalities: Condoms, Coups, and

the Ideology of Prevention: Facing Failure in Rural Haiti," in *Catholic Ethicists on HIV/AIDS Prevention*, 118.

42. Ibid., 119. Many of these claims have been refuted. See, for example, Farmer, "Medicine and Social Justice," and Tina Rosenberg, "Look at Brazil," *New York Times Magazine*, 28 January 2001, 26.

43. Kidder, "The Good Doctor," 42.

44. Ibid., 44.

45. Ibid., 56–57. At another point Farmer's answer to "what does it mean to be human" is "solidarity, compassion, sympathy, and love" (57).

46. Ibid., 57.

47. Ibid., 56.

48. Ibid.

Conclusion

1. We would do well to even begin with *The Catholic Common Ground Initiative* listing of principles for dialogue at http://www.nplc.org/commonground/dialogue.htm. See also the five elements of a "spirituality of dialogue" that John L. Allen Jr. recently offered (epistemological humility; solid formation in Catholic tradition, as a means of creating a common language; patience; perspective—the capacity to see issues through the eyes of others; healthy assertion of Catholic identity). The text is available at http://www.ncronline.org/mainpage/specialdocuments/allen_common.htm.

2. If you have a success story to share (your own or that of another), please send it with your full name and email address to mcimperman@ost.edu. Please write under the subject heading AIDS Success Story. A website will soon be created to share the stories more widely. Permission to share the stories will be presumed unless you indicate otherwise. Thank you!

Selected Bibliography

Ackermann, Denise M. "'Deep in the Flesh': Women, Bodies and HIV/AIDS: Feminist Ethical Perspective" (manuscript sent from South Africa).
———. "Reconciliation as Embodied Change: A South African Perspective." *Proceedings of the Catholic Theological Society of America* 59 (2004): 50–67. "AIDS Finally Is Described by the Chinese as Epidemic." *New York Times*, 17 December 2000, NE5.
Alarcon, Jorge O., Kay M. Johnson, Barry Courtois, Carlos Rodriguez, Jorge Sanchez, Douglas M. Watts, and King K. Holmes. "Determinants and Prevalence of HIV Infection in Pregnant Peruvian Women." *AIDS* 17 (2003): 613–18.
Andolsen, Barbara Hilkert. "Agape in Feminist Ethics." *Journal of Religious Ethics* 9.1 (Spring 1981): 69–83.
———. "Whose Sexuality? Whose Tradition? Women, Experience and Roman Catholic Catholic Sexual Ethics." In *Religion and Sexual Health: Ethical, Theological, and Clinical Perspectives*. Edited by Ronald M. Green, 55–77. Boston: Kluwer Academic Publishers, 1992.
Aquinas, Saint Thomas. *Introduction to Saint Thomas Aquinas*. Edited by Anton C. Pegis. New York: The Modern Library, 1945; Random House, 1948.
———. *St. Thomas Aquinas on Politics and Ethics: A New Translation, Backgrounds, Interpretations*. Translated and edited by Paul E. Sigmund. New York: W. W. Norton & Company, 1988.
———. *Treatise on the Virtues*. Translated by John A. Oesterle. Englewood Cliffs, NJ: Prentice-Hall, 1966; Reprint, University of Notre Dame Press, 1984.
Arellano, Luz Beatriz. "Women's Experience of God in Emerging Spirituality." In *Feminist Theology from the Third World: A Reader*. Edited by Ursula King, 318–38. New York: SPCK/Orbis, 1994.
Aristotle. *Nicomachean Ethics*. Translated by Martin Ostwald. Englewood Cliffs, NJ: Prentice Hall, 1962.
Ashley, James Matthew. *Interruptions: Mysticism, Politics, and Theology in the Work of Johann Baptist Metz*. Notre Dame, IN: University of Notre Dame Press, 1998.
Beauchamp, Tom L. "What's So Special about the Virtues?" In *Virtue and Medicine: Explorations in the Character of Medicine*. Edited by Earl E. Shelp. *Philosophy and Medicine* 17, Dordrecht, the Netherlands: D. Reidel Publishing, 1985.
Beauchamp, Tom L., and James F. Childress. *Principles of Biomedical Ethics*, 3rd ed. New York: Oxford University Press, 2001.
Bednar, Gerald J. *Faith as Imagination: The Contribution of William F. Lynch, S.J.* Kansas City: Sheed & Ward, 1996.

Bilgrien, Marie Vianney, SSND. *Solidarity: A Principle, an Attitude, a Duty? or the Virtue for an Interdependent World?* New York: Peter Lang Publishing, 1999.

Billy, Dennis. "Aquinas on the Relations of Prudence." *Studia Moralia* 33 (1995): 250.

Boff, Leonardo. *When Theology Listens to the Poor.* San Francisco: Harper & Row, 1988.

Bonhoeffer, Dietrich. *The Cost of Discipleship.* New York: Macmillan, 1959.

Bourke-Martignoni, Joanna. *Violence against Women in Zambia: Report Prepared for the Committee on the Elimination of Discrimination against Women.* Available at http://www.omct/pdf/vaw/zambiaeng2002.pdf. Internet. Accessed 7 September 2004.

Bradshaw, John. *Bradshaw on the Family: A New Way of Creating Self-Esteem*, rev. ed. Deerfield Beach, FL: Health Communications, 1996.

Braxton, Joanne M. *Black Women Writing Autobiography: A Tradition Within a Tradition.* Philadelphia: Temple University Press, 1988.

Brueggemann, Walter. *Hopeful Imagination: Prophetic Voices in Exile.* Philadelphia: Fortress Press, 1986.

Burggraeve, Roger. "From Responsible to Meaningful Sexuality: An Ethics of Growth as an Ethics of Mercy for Young People in This Era of AIDS." In *Catholic Ethicists on HIV/AIDS Prevention.* Edited by James F. Keenan, assisted by Jon D. Fuller, Lisa Sowle Cahill, and Kevin Kelly, 303–16. New York: Continuum, 2000.

———. *From Self-Development to Solidarity: An Ethical Reading of Human Desire in Its Socio-Political Relevance According to Emmanuel Levinas.* Grand Rapids, MI: Peeters Publishers, 1985.

———. "Prohibition and Taste: The Bipolarity in Christian Ethics." *Ethical Perspectives* 1, no. 3 (1994): 130–44.

———. "Une Ethique de miséricorde." *Lumen Vitae: Revue internationale de caté-chèse et de pastorale* 49 (September 1994): 281–96.

Burggraeve, Roger, and Marc Vervenne. *Swords into Plowshares: Theological Reflections on Peace.* Louvain Theological and Pastoral Monographs 8. Grand Rapids, MI: Peeters Publishers, 1991.

Burke, Kevin F. *The Ground Beneath the Cross: The Theology of Ignacio Ellacuría.* Washington, DC: Georgetown University Press, 2000.

Cahill, Lisa Sowle. "AIDS, Justice and the Common Good." In *Catholic Ethicists on HIV/AIDS Prevention.* Edited by James F. Keenan, assisted by Jon D. Fuller, Lisa Sowle Cahill, and Kevin Kelly, 282–88. New York: Continuum, 2000.

———. *Between the Sexes: Foundations for a Christian Ethics of Sexuality.* Philadelphia: Fortress Press, 1985.

———. *Gender and Christian Ethics.* Cambridge: Cambridge University Press, 1996.

———. *Humanity as Female and Male: The Ethics of Sexuality.* Edited by Francis A. Eigo. Villanova, PA: Villanova University Press, 1985.

———. "Marriage: Developments in Catholic Theology and Ethics." *Theological Studies* 64 (2003): 78–105.

———. " 'Embodiment' and Moral Critique: A Christian Social Perspective." In *Embodiment, Morality and Medicine.* Edited by Lisa Sowle Cahill and Margaret A. Farley. Boston: Kluwer Academic Publishers, 1995, 199–215.

Carabine, Deirdre, and Martin O'Reilly, eds. "The Challenge of Eradicating Poverty in the World: An African Response." *Proceedings of the International Conference held at Uganda Martyrs University, Nkozi, 7–10 September 1998.* Nkozi: Uganda Martyrs University Press.

"Cardinal Ratzinger's Letter on AIDS Document." *Origins* 18.8 (1988): 117–21.

Carl, Maria. "Law, Virtue, and Happiness in Aquinas' Moral Theory." *Thomist* 61 (1997): 427.

Cassell, Eric J. *The Nature of Suffering and the Goals of Medicine.* New York: Oxford University Press, 1991.

Catechism of the Catholic Church. New York: Doubleday, 1995. First Image Books, 1995.

Cates, Diana Fritz. *Choosing to Feel: Virtue, Friendship, and Compassion for Friends.* Notre Dame, IN: University of Notre Dame Press, 1997.

Catholic Biblical Association of America, Confraternity of Christian Doctrine, and Bishops' Committee. *New American Bible.* New York: P. J. Kenedy, 1970.

"Caution Greets AIDS Statement by French Bishops." *The Tablet*, 24 February 1996, 256–57.

Cessario, Romanus. "The Theological Virtue of Hope." In *The Ethics of Aquinas.* Edited by Stephen J. Pope, 232–43. Washington, DC: Georgetown University Press, 2002.

Chopp, Rebecca S. "Praxis." In *The New Dictionary of Catholic Spirituality.* Edited by Michael Downey, 756–64. Collegeville, MN: Liturgical Press, 1993.

———. *The Praxis of Suffering: An Interpretation of Liberation and Political Theologies.* Maryknoll, NY: Orbis Books, 1986.

"The Church and Condoms." *The Southern Cross.* 10 December 2002, 4.

"Church Leaders Mix Condoms and Caveats." *National Catholic Reporter*, 15 March 1996.

Clarke, Katherine M. "Lessons from Feminist Therapy for Ministerial Ethics." *Journal of Pastoral Care* 48 (1994): 233–42.

Clifford, Anne M. *Introducing Feminist Theology.* Maryknoll, NY: Orbis Books, 2001.

Coll, Regina A. *Christianity and Feminism in Conversation.* Mystic, CT: Twenty-Third Publications, 1994.

Collins, Raymond F. *Sexual Ethics and the New Testament: Behavior and Belief.* New York: Crossroad, 2000.

"The Condom Debate." *The Southern Cross.* 18 July 2001.

Congregation for the Doctrine of the Faith. "Declaration on Certain Questions Concerning Sexual Ethics." *(Persona humana).* 29 December 1975. In *Vatican Council II: More Postconciliar Documents.* Edited by Austin Flannery, 77–96. Grand Rapids, MI: Eerdmans, 1982.

Connors, Russell B., Jr., and Patrick T. McCormick. *Character, Choices & Community: The Three Faces of Christian Ethics.* New York: Paulist Press, 1998.

Cooper, Helene, Rachel Zimmerman, and Laurie McGinley. "AIDS Epidemic Puts Drug Firms in a Vise: Treatment vs. Profits." *Wall Street Journal*, 2 March 2001. Available at http://interactive.wsj.com/articles/SB983487988418159849.htm.

Copeland, M. Shawn. " 'Wading Through Many Sorrows': Toward a Theology of Suffering in Womanist Perspective." In *Feminist Ethics and the Catholic Moral Tradition.* Edited by Charles E. Curran, Margaret A. Farley, and Richard A. McCormick, 36–163. New York: Paulist Press, 1996.

Crosby, Michael H., OFM, Cap. "Justice." In *The New Dictionary of Catholic Spirituality.* Edited by Michael Downey, 578–83. Collegeville, MN: Liturgical Press, 1993.

Cunningham, Lawrence S., and Keith J. Egan. *Christian Spirituality: Themes from the Tradition.* New York: Paulist Press, 1996.

Curran, Charles E. *The Catholic Moral Tradition Today: A Synthesis.* Washington, DC: Georgetown University Press, 1999.

———. *Moral Theology: A Continuing Journey.* Notre Dame, IN: University of Notre Dame Press, 1982.

Curran, Charles E., ed. *Moral Theology: Challenges for the Future. Essays in Honor of Richard A. McCormick.* New York: Paulist Press, 1990.

Curran, Charles E., Margaret A. Farley, and Richard A. McCormick, SJ, eds. *Feminist Ethics and the Catholic Moral Tradition.* New York: Paulist Press, 1996.

De los Pando, M., et al. "High Human Immunodeficiency Virus Type 1 Seroprevalence in Men Who Have Sex with Men in Buenos Aires, Argentina: Risk Factors for Infection. *International Journal of Epidemiology* 32 (2003): 735–40.

Demmer, Klaus, MSC. *Shaping the Moral Life: An Approach to Moral Theology.* Edited by James F. Keenan, SJ, with a foreword by Thomas Kopfensteiner. Translated by Roberto Dell'Oro. Washington, DC: Georgetown University Press, 2000.

Demmer, Klaus. "La competenza normativa del magistero ecclesiastico in morale." In *Fede cristiana e agire morale.* Edited by Klaus Demmer and Bruno Schuller, 144–71. Assisi: Cittadella editrice, 1980.

Diaz, T., S. Y. Chu, J. W. Buehler, D. Boyd, P. J. Checko, L. Conti, A. J. Davidson, P. Hermann, M. Herr, A. Levy, et al. "Socioeconomic Differences among People with AIDS: Results from a Multistate Surveillance Project." *American Journal of Preventive Medicine* 10, no. 4 (1994): 217–22.

Dietrich, Bonhoeffer. *The Cost of Discipleship.* New York: Macmillan, 1959.

Donnelly, John. "Deal on AIDS Drugs Fuels Push for More Funds: Indian Firm Agrees to Provide Treatment Cheaply to Charity." *Boston Globe,* 8 February 2001.

Dorr, Donal. *Option for the Poor: A Hundred Years of Catholic Social Teaching,* rev. ed. Maryknoll, NY: Orbis Books, 1983, 1992.

———. *Spirituality and Justice.* Maryknoll, NY: Orbis Books, 1984.

Downey, Michael, ed. *The New Dictionary of Catholic Spirituality.* Collegeville, MN: Liturgical Press, 1993.

Drane, James. "Condoms, AIDS, and Catholic Ethics." *Commonweal* 189 (1991): 188–92.

Drinan, Robert F. *The Mobilization of Shame: A World View of Human Rights.* New Haven, CT: Yale University Press, 2001.

"Dutch Cardinal Says Condoms OK When Spouse Has AIDS." *Catholic News Service,* 16 February 1996.

Eberstadt, Nicholas. "The Future of AIDS." *Foreign Affairs* 81, no. 6 (2002): 22–45.

Ekkehard, Schuster, and Reinhold Boschert-Kimmig. *Hope Against Hope: Johann Baptist Metz and Elie Wiesel Speak Out on the Holocaust.* Translated by J. Matthew Ashley. New York: Paulist Press, 1999.

Ela, Jean-Marc. "Christianity and Liberation in Africa." In *Paths of African Theology.* Edited by Rosino Gibellini, 136–53. Maryknoll, NY: Orbis Books, 1994.

Ela, Jean-Marc. *African Cry.* Translated by Robert R. Barr. Maryknoll, NY: Orbis Books, 1986.

Ellacuría, Ignacio. "The Crucified People." In *Mysterium Liberationis: Fundamental Concepts of Liberation Theology.* Edited by Ignatio Ellacuria and Jon Sobrino, 580–603. Maryknoll, NY: Orbis Books, 1993.

Empereur, James L., SJ, and Christopher G. Kiesling, OP. *The Liturgy That Does Justice.* Collegeville, MN: Liturgical Press, 1990.

Fabella, Virginia, M. M., and Mercy Amba Oduyoye, eds., *With Passion and Compassion: Third World Women Doing Theology*. Maryknoll, NY: Orbis Books, 1988.

Farley, Margaret A. "Compassionate Respect: A Feminist Approach to Medical Ethics and Other Questions." *2002 Madeleva Lecture in Spirituality*. New York: Paulist Press, 2002.

———. "Feminism and Universal Morality." In *Prospects for a Common Morality*. Edited by G. Outka and J. Reeder, 170–90. Princeton, NJ: Princeton University Press, 1993.

———. "A Feminist Version of Respect for Persons." *Journal of Feminist Studies in Religion* 9 (Spring/Fall, 1993): 182–98. Reprinted in *Feminist Ethics and the Catholic Moral Tradition*. Edited by Charles E. Curran, Margaret A. Farley, and Richard McCormick, 164–83. Mahwah, NJ: Paulist Press, 1996.

———. "Fragments for an Ethic of Commitment in Thomas Aquinas." In *Celebrating the Medieval Heritage. Journal of Religion* 58, Suppl. (1978): 40–45.

———. "How Shall We Love in a Postmodern World?" *The Annual of the Society of Christian Ethics*. Washington, DC: Georgetown University Press, 1994.

———. "New Patterns of Relationship Between Women and Men: The Beginnings of a Moral Revolution," *Theological Studies* 36 (December 1975): 627–46. Reprinted in *Woman: New Dimensions*. Edited by Walter Burkhardt, 51–70. New York: Paulist Press, 1975.

———. *Personal Commitments: Beginning, Keeping, Changing*. San Francisco: Harper & Row, 1986.

———. "Sources of Sexual Inequality in the History of Christian Thought." *Journal of Religion* 56 (April 1976): 163–69.

Farmer, Paul. *Infections and Inequalities: The Modern Plagues*. Berkeley, CA: University of California Press, 1999, 2001.

———. "Medicine and Social Justice." *America* 173, no. 2 (15 July 1995): 13–17.

———. "Prevention Without Treatment Is Not Sustainable." *National AIDS Bulletin* (Australia) 13, no. 6 (2000): 6–7.

———. "Women, Poverty, and AIDS." In *Women, Poverty, and AIDS: Sex, Drugs, and Structural Violence*. Edited by Paul Farmer, Maureen Connors, and Janie Simmons. Monroe, ME: Common Courage Press, 1996.

Farmer, Paul and David Walton. "Revealing and Critiquing Inequalities: Condoms, Coups, and the Ideology of Prevention: Facing Failure in Rural Haiti." In *Catholic Ethicists on HIV/AIDS Prevention*. Edited by James F. Keenan, assisted by Jon D. Fuller, Lisa Sowle Cahill, and Kevin Kelly, 108–19. New York: Continuum, 2000.

Farmer, Paul, M. Connors, and J. Simmons, eds. *Women, Poverty, and AIDS: Sex Drugs, and Structural Violence*. Monroe, ME: Common Courage Press, 1996.

Ferder, Fran, and John Heagle. *Tender Fires: The Spiritual Promise of Sexuality*. New York: Crossroad, 2002.

———. *Your Sexual Self: Pathway to Authentic Intimacy*. Notre Dame, IN: Ave Maria, 1992.

Ferrer, Jorge J. "Needle Exchange in San Juan, Puerto Rico: A Traditional Roman Catholic Casuistic Approach." In *Catholic Ethicists on HIV/AIDS Prevention*. Edited by James F. Keenan, assisted by Jon D. Fuller, Lisa Sowle Cahill, and Kevin Kelly, 177–91. New York: Continuum, 2000.

Fiorenza, Elisabeth Schussler. *Discipleship of Equals: A Critical Feminist Ekklesialogy of Liberation*. New York: Crossroad, 1993.

Fiorenza, Francis P. "Political Theology and Liberation Theology: An Inquiry into Their Fundamental Meaning." In *Liberation, Revolution, and Freedom: Theological Perspectives. Proceedings of the College Theology Society.* Edited by Thomas M. McFadden, 3–29. New York: Crossroad, 1975.

Flannery, Austin, ed. *Vatican Council II: More Postconciliar Documents*, English ed. Grand Rapids, MI: Eerdmans, 1982.

Flynn, Eileen P. *Catholicism: Agenda For Renewal.* Lanham, MD: University Press of America, 1994.

———. "Teaching about HIV Prevention in an American Catholic College Classroom." In *Catholic Ethicists on HIV/AIDS Prevention.* Edited by James F. Keenan, assisted by Jon D. Fuller, Lisa Sowle Cahill, and Kevin Kelly, 148–54. New York: Continuum, 2000.

Flynn, Raymond, and Robin Moore. *The Accidental Pope.* New York: St. Martin's Press, 2000.

Freire, Paulo. *Pedagogy of the Oppressed*, new rev. 20th anniversary ed. Translated by Myra Bergman Ramos. New York: Continuum, 1997.

Fuller, Jon. "AIDS and the Church: A Stimulus to Our Theologizing." Lecture given at Weston Jesuit School of Theology, Boston, Mass., 12 March 1991.

———. "AIDS Prevention: A Challenge to the Catholic Moral Tradition." *America* 175 (28 December 1996): 13–20.

———. "Needle Exchange: Saving Lives." *America* 179 (18–25 July 1998): 8–11.

Fuller, Jon D., and James F. Keenan. "Introduction: At the End of the First Generation of HIV Prevention." In *Catholic Ethicists on HIV/AIDS Prevention.* Edited by James F. Keenan, assisted by Jon D. Fuller, Lisa Sowle Cahill, and Kevin Kelly, 21–38. New York: Continuum, 2000.

———. "Condoms, Catholics and HIV/AIDS Prevention." *The Furrow* 52, no. 9 (Sept. 2001): 459–67.

———. "Church Politics and HIV Prevention: Why Is the Condom Question So Significant and So Neuralgic?" *Between Poetry and Politics: Essays in Honour of Enda McDonagh.* Edited by Barbara Fitzgerald and Linda Hogan, 158–81. Dublin: Columba Press, 2003.

Gallagher, Joseph. *Voices of Strength and Hope for a Friend with AIDS.* Kansas City, MO: Sheed & Ward, 1987.

Gebara, Ivone. "Women Doing Theology in Latin America." In *Liberation Theology: An Introductory Reader.* Edited by Curt Cardorette, Marie Giblin, Marilyn J. Legge, and Mary H. Snyder, 56–63. Maryknoll, NY: Orbis Books, 1992.

Genovesi, Vincent J., SJ. *Expectant Creativity: The Action of Hope in Christian Ethics.* Lanham, MD: University Press of America, 1982.

———. *In Pursuit of Love: Catholic Morality and Human Sexuality*, 2d ed. Collegeville, MN: Liturgical Press, 1996.

Gibellini, Rosino, ed. *Paths of African Theology.* Maryknoll, NY: Orbis Books, 1994.

Goizueta, Roberto S. *Caminemos con Jesús: Toward a Hispanic/Latino Theology of Accompaniment.* Maryknoll, NY: Orbis Books, 1995.

———. "Solidarity." In *New Dictionary of Catholic Spirituality.* Edited by Michael Downey, 906. Collegeville, MN: Liturgical Press, 1993.

Gramick, Jennine, and Robert Nugent, eds. *Voices of Hope.* New York: Center for Homophobia Education, 1995.

Gravato, N., M. G. G. Morell, K. Areco, and C. A. Peres. "Associated Factors to

HIV Infection in Commercial Sex Workers in Santos, Sao Paulo, Brazil." XV International AIDS Conference, Bangkok, 11–16 July 2004. Abstract WePeC6162.

Green, Ronald M., ed. *Religion and Sexual Health: Ethical, Theological, and Clinical Perspectives.* Dordrecht, the Netherlands: Kluwer Academic Publishers, 1992.

Guanira, J. et al. "Second Generation of HIV Surveillance among Men Who Have Sex with Men in Peru during 2002." XV International AIDS Conference, Bangkok, 11–16 July 2004. Abstract WePeC6162.

Gudorf, Christine. *Body, Sex and Pleasure: Reconstructing Christian Sexual Ethics.* Cleveland, OH: Pilgrim Press, 1994.

Gula, Richard M., SS. *The Call to Holiness: Embracing a Fully Christian Life.* New York: Paulist Press, 2003.

———. *The Good Life: Where Morality and Spirituality Converge.* New York: Paulist Press, 1999.

———. *Moral Discernment.* New York: Paulist Press, 1997.

———. *Reason Informed by Faith: Foundations of Catholic Morality.* New York: Paulist Press, 1989.

Gutiérrez, Gustavo. *A Theology of Liberation: History, Politics, and Salvation,* rev. ed. with a new Introduction. Translated and edited by Sister Caridad Inda and John Eagleson. Maryknoll, NY: Orbis Books, 1988.

———. *The Density of the Present: Selected Writings.* Maryknoll, NY: Orbis Books, 1999.

———. *We Drink from Our Own Wells: The Spiritual Journey of a People.* Translated by Matthew J. O'Connell. Maryknoll, NY: Orbis Books, 1984.

Guttmacher, Sally, Lisa Lieberman, and David Ward. "Does Access to Condoms Influence Adolescent Sexual Behavior?" *The AIDS Reader* 8 (November/December 1998): 201–205, 209.

Haight, Roger. *The Experience and Language of Grace.* New York: Paulist Press, 1979.

Hamel, Ronald P., and Kenneth R. Himes, eds. *Introduction to Christian Ethics: A Reader.* New York: Paulist Press, 1989.

Hampshire, Stuart. *Thought and Action.* Notre Dame, IN: University of Notre Dame Press, 1983.

Hanigan, James P. *What Are They Saying About Sexual Morality?* New York: Paulist Press, 1982.

Häring, Bernard. *The Law of Christ.* Westminster, MD: Newman Press, 1961.

———. *The Virtues of an Authentic Life: A Celebration of Spiritual Maturity.* Translated by Peter Heinegg. Liguori, MO: Liguori, 1997.

Häring, Bernard, and Valentino Salvoldi. *Tolerance: Towards an Ethic of Solidarity and Peace.* Translated by Edmund C. Lane, SSP. New York: Alba House, 1995.

Harrington, Daniel J., SJ. *Why Do We Suffer: A Scriptural Approach to the Human Condition.* Franklin, WI: Sheed & Ward, 2000.

Harrington, Daniel J., SJ, and James F. Keenan, SJ. *Jesus and Virtue Ethics: Building Bridges Between New Testament Studies and Moral Theology.* Lanham, MD: Sheed & Ward, 2002.

Harvey, Nicholas Peter. "Listening in England to a Woman's Life Experience." In *Catholic Ethicists on HIV/AIDS Prevention.* Edited by James F. Keenan, assisted by Jon D. Fuller, Lisa Sowle Cahill, and Kevin Kelly, 70–75. New York: Continuum, 2000.

Hauerwas, Stanley. *A Community of Character: Toward a Constructive Christian Social Ethic*. Notre Dame, IN: University of Notre Dame Press, 1981.

Hays, Richard B. *The Moral Vision of the New Testament: Community, Cross, New Creation*. San Francisco: HarperSan Francisco, 1996.

Henry J. Kaiser Family Foundation. "The Global HIV/AIDS Epidemic," *HIV/AIDS Policy Fact Sheet*. December 2004. Available at http://www.kff.org. Internet. Accessed 12 December 2004.

Hilkert, Mary Catherine. *Naming Grace: Preaching and the Sacramental Imagination*. New York: Continuum, 1997.

———. "Speaking with Authority: Catherine of Siena and the Voices of Women Today." *2001 Madeleva Lecture in Spirituality*. New York: Paulist Press, 2001.

Hinsdale, Mary Ann. "Heeding the Voices: An Historical Overview." In *In The Embrace of God: Feminist Approaches to Theological Anthropology*. Edited by Ann O'Hara Graff, 22–38. Maryknoll, NY: Orbis Books, 1995.

Hogan, Linda. *Confronting the Truth: Conscience in the Catholic Tradition*. New York: Paulist Press, 2000.

———. "An Irish Nun Living with Contradictions: Responding to HIV/AIDS in the Context of Church Teaching." In *Catholic Ethicists on HIV/AIDS Prevention*. Edited by James F. Keenan, assisted by Jon D. Fuller, Lisa Sowle Cahill, and Kevin Kelly, 41–47. New York: Continuum, 2000.

Hollenbach, David. *The Common Good and Christian Ethics*. New York: Cambridge University Press, 2002.

———. *The Common Good in a Divided Society*. Santa Clara, CA: Santa Clara University, 1999; New York: Cambridge University Press, 2002.

Iozzio, Mary Jo. *Self-Determination and the Moral Act: A Study of the Contributions of Odon Lottin (OSB)*. Grand Rapids, MI: Peeters Publishers, 1995.

Isasi-Díaz, Ada María. *Mujerista Theology: A Theology for the Twenty-First Century*. Maryknoll, NY: Orbis Books, 1996.

———. "Solidarity: Love of Neighbor in the 1980s." In *Lift Every Voice: Constructing Christian Theologies from the Underside*. Edited by Susan Brooks Thistlethwaite and Mary Potter Engel, 31–39. San Francisco: Harper & Row, 1990.

Janssens, Louis. "Artificial Insemination: Ethical Considerations." *Louvain Studies* 8. In *Reason Informed by Faith: Foundations of Catholic Morality*. Edited by Richard M. Gula, SS, 3–29. New York: Paulist Press, 1989.

Johnson, Elizabeth A. *Consider Jesus: Waves of Renewal in Christology*. New York: Crossroad, 1990.

———. "Jesus and Salvation." *Proceedings of the Catholic Theological Society of America* 49 (1994): 1–18.

———. *She Who Is: The Mystery of God in Feminist Theological Discourse*. New York: Crossroad, 1992.

Johnson, K. M., Jorge Alarcon, Douglas M. Watts, Carlos Rodriguez, Carlos Valasquez, Jorge Sanchez, David Lockhart, Bradley P. Stoner, and King K. Holmes. "Sexual Networks of Pregnant Women with and without HIV Infection." *AIDS* 17, no. 4 (2003): 605–12; UNAIDS/WHO, *AIDS Epidemic Update: December 2004*, 58.

Joint United Nations Programme on HIV/AIDS (UNAIDS). *AIDS Epidemic Update: December 2002*. Available at www.unaids.org.

———. "Fact Sheets—Men Make a Difference" [data online]. Available at http://www.unaids.org/fact_sheets/ files/WAC_Eng.html.

———. *Gender and HIV/AIDS: Taking Stock of Research and Programmes.* Geneva, 1999.

———. "Have You Heard Me Today?" *World AIDS Campaign on Women and Girls.* Available at http://www.unaids.org/wac2004/index_en.htm. Internet. Accessed 27 December 2004.

———. *Report on the Global HIV/AIDS Epidemic—AIDS in a New Millennium, 2000* [report online]. Available at www.unaids.org/epidemic_update/report/ Epi_report_chap_millenium.htm. Internet.

———. *Report on the Global HIV/AIDS Epidemic, 2002* [report online]. Available at www.unaids.org/barcelona/presskit/barcelona%20report/preface.html. Internet. Accessed 10 October 2002.

Joint United Nations Programme on HIV/AIDS (UNAIDS) and World Health Organization. *2000 AIDS Epidemic Update: December 2000* [report online]. Available at www.unaids.org/epidemic_update/report/epi_core/sld001.htm. Internet. Accessed March 2001.

———. *AIDS Epidemic Update: December 2004*, 2. Available at http://www.unaids.org/wad2004/ EPI_1204_pdf_en/EpiUpdate04_en.pdf. Internet. Accessed 27 November 2004.

———. *2004 Report on the Global HIV/AIDS Epidemic, July 2004* [report on line]. See http://www.unaids.org.

———. "Summary Report, National HIV and Syphilis Sero-Prevalence Survey of Women Attending Public Antenatal Clinics in South Africa, 2001." Department of Health, South Africa. Available at www.unaids.org.

———. "Women and AIDS—A Growing Challenge." Fact Sheet. Available at http://www.unaids.org/html/pub/publications/fact-sheets04/FS_Women_en_pdf. Internet. Accessed 9 December 2004.

Jung, Patricia. "Sanctification: An Interpretation in Light of Embodiment." *Journal of Religious Ethics* 11 (1983): 75–94.

Kaleeba, Noerine. Address to the World Health Assembly, May 2001. Available at www.unaids.org/whatsnew/speeches/eng/kaleeba1405who.htm.

———. Quoted in "Profile: International Dream Team: She's the One." In *Pox: Health, Hope and HIV.* Cited in website: www.poxy.com in July 1998.

———. "Stigma and AIDS." Keynote address. Available at http://www.hdnet.org/ Stigma/Meeting%20Agenda%20and%20presentations/Keynote%20address.htm.

———. *We Miss You All.* Harare, Zimbabwe: Women and AIDS Support Network, 1991.

Kaleeba, Noerine, Joyce Namulondo Kadowe, Daniel Kalinaki, and Glen Williams. "Open Secret: People Facing Up to HIV and AIDS in Uganda." In *Strategies for Hope Series,* no. 15. London: ACTIONAID, 2000.

Kaleeba, Noerine, Sunanda Ray, and Brigid Willmore. *We Miss You All: AIDS in the Family.* Kampala, Uganda: Marianum Press, 1993.

Kalilombe, Patrick A. "Spirituality in the African Perspective." In *Paths of African Theology.* Edited by Rosino Gibellini, 115–35. Maryknoll, NY: Orbis Books, 1994.

Keane, Philip, SS. *Christian Ethics and Imagination: A Theological Inquiry.* New York: Paulist Press, 1984.

———. *Sexual Morality: A Catholic Perspective.* New York: Paulist Press, 1977.

Keating, James, ed. *Spirituality and Moral Theology: Essays from a Pastoral Perspective.* New York: Paulist Press, 2000.

Keenan, James F., SJ. "Christian Perspectives on the Human Body." *Theological Studies* 55 (June 1994): 330–46.

———. *Commandments of Compassion.* Franklin, WI: Sheed & Ward, 1999.

———. "Dualism in Medicine, Christian Theology, and the Aging." *Journal of Religion and Health* 35 (1996): 3–46.

———. "Ethics and Spirituality: Historical Distinctions and Contemporary Challenges," *Listening* (Fall 1999): 167–79.

———. *Goodness and Rightness in Thomas Aquinas's Summa Theologiae.* Washington, DC: Georgetown University Press, 1992.

———. "How Catholic Are the Virtues?" *America* 176, no. 20 (June 1997): 16–22.

———. "The Moral Agent: Actions and Normative Decision-Making." In *A Call to Fidelity: On the Moral Theology of Charles E. Curran.* Edited by James J. Walter, Timothy E. O'Connell, and Thomas A. Shannon, 41. Washington, DC: Georgetown University Press, 2002.

———. "The Open Debate: Moral Theology and the Lives of Gay and Lesbian Persons." *Theological Studies* 64 (2003): 127–50.

———. *Practice What You Preach: The Need for Ethics in Church Leadership.* Annual Jesuit Lecture in Human Values. Milwaukee: Marquette University, 2000.

———. "Prophylactics, Toleration and Cooperation: Contemporary Moral Problems and Traditional Principles." *International Philosophical Quarterly* 28 (1988): 201–20.

———. "Proposing Cardinal Virtues." *Theological Studies* 56 (1995): 708–29.

———. "The Return of Casuistry." *Theological Studies* 57 (1996): 123–39.

———. "Spirituality and Morality: What's the Difference?" In *Method and Catholic Moral Theology: The Ongoing Reconstruction.* Edited by Todd A. Salzman, 87–102. Omaha, NE: Creighton University Press, 1999.

———. "Virtue and Identity." *Concilium* 2 (2000): 69–75.

———. "Virtue Ethics." In *Christian Ethics: An Introduction.* Edited by Bernard Hoose, 89–94. Collegeville, MN: Liturgical Press, 1998.

———. *Virtues for Ordinary Christians.* Franklin, WI: Sheed & Ward, 1999.

———. "The Virtue of Prudence (IIa IIae, qq 47–56)." In *The Ethics of Aquinas.* Edited by Stephen J. Pope, 259–71. Washington, DC: Georgetown University Press, 2002.

Keenan, James F., ed. *Catholic Ethicists on HIV/AIDS Prevention.* Assisted by Jon D. Fuller, Lisa Sowle Cahill, and Kevin Kelly. New York: Continuum, 2000.

Keenan, James F., and Thomas Kopfensteiner. "The Principle of Material Cooperation." *Health Progress* 76.3 (April 1995): 23–27.

Kelly, Kevin T. "Conclusion: A Moral Theologian Faces the New Millennium in a Time of AIDS." In *Catholic Ethicists on HIV/AIDS Prevention.* Edited by James F. Keenan, assisted by Jon D. Fuller, Lisa Sowle Cahill, and Kevin Kelly, 324–32. New York: Continuum, 2000.

———. *New Directions in Sexual Ethics: Moral Theology and the Challenge of AIDS.* London and Washington, DC: Geoffrey Chapman, 1998.

———. *New Directions in Moral Theology: The Challenge of Being Human.* London: Geoffrey Chapman, 1992.

Kidder, Tracy. "The Good Doctor." *New Yorker*, 10 July 2000, 42, 44, 56–57.

————. *Mountains Beyond Mountains: The Quest of Dr. Paul Farmer, A Man Who Would Cure the World.* New York: Random House: 2003.

Kim, Jim Yong, Joyce V. Millen, Alec Irwin, and John Gershman, eds. *Dying for Growth: Global Inequality and the Health of the Poor.* Monroe, ME: Common Courage Press, 2000.

King, Ursula, ed. *Feminist Theology from the Third World: A Reader.* New York/London: SPCK/Orbis Books, 1994.

Kirby, Douglas, Nancy D. Brener, Ron Harrist, N. Peterfreund, and P. Hillard. "The Impact of Condom Distribution in Seattle Schools on Sexual Behavior and Condom Use." *American Journal of Public Health* 89 (February 1999): 182–87.

Kotva, Joseph J. *The Christian Case for Virtue Ethics.* Washington, DC: Georgetown University Press, 1996.

LaCugna, Catherine M. *God for Us: The Trinity and Christian Life.* San Francisco: Harper, 1991.

LaCugna, Catherine Mowry, ed. *Freeing Theology: The Essentials of Theology in Feminist Perspective.* San Francisco: Harper, 1993.

La Documentation Catholique, no. 2176. (1998): 191–95.

Lane, Belden C. "Narrative." In *New Dictionary of Catholic Spirituality.* Edited by Michael Downey, 696. Collegeville, MN: Liturgical Press, 1993.

Lauritzen, Paul. "Emotions and Religious Ethics." *Journal of Religious Ethics* 16 (1988): 307–24.

Lawler, Ronald Joseph Boyle, Jr., and William E. May. *Catholic Sexual Ethics: A Summary, Explanation, & Defense,* 2nd ed. Huntington, IN: Our Sunday Visitor, 1998.

Lebacqz, Karen. "Appropriate Vulnerability: A Sexual Ethic for Singles." *The Christian Century* 104, no. 15 (6 May 1987): 435–38.

————. *Justice in an Unjust World: Foundations For A Christian Approach To Justice.* Minneapolis, MN: Augsburg Publishing House, 1987.

————. "Justice." In *Christian Ethics: An Introduction.* Edited by Bernard Hoose, 163–72. Collegeville, MN: Liturgical Press, 1998.

————. *Six Theories of Justice: Perspectives from Philosophical and Theological Ethics.* Minneapolis, MN: Augsburg Publishing House, 1986.

Lohfink, Norbert F., S.J. *Option for the Poor: The Basic Principle of Liberation Theology in the Light of the Bible.* Edited by Duane L. Christensen. Translated by Linda M. Maloney, Ph.D. North Richland Hills, TX: BIBAL Press, 1987; 2nd ed., 1995.

Lonsdale, David. *Eyes to See, Ears to Hear.* Chicago: Loyola University Press, 1990.

Lumen Vitae: Revue internationale de catéchèse et de pastorale 49 (September 1994): 281–96.

Lynch, William F., S.J. *Images of Hope: Imagination as Healer of the Hopeless.* Baltimore: Helicon Press, 1965.

MacIntyre, Alasdair. *After Virtue.* Notre Dame, IN: University of Notre Dame Press, 1988.

Macnamara, Vincent. "The Moral Journey." *The Way* 88, Suppl. (Spring 1997): 6–15.

Madigan, Shawn. *Spirituality Rooted in Liturgy,* rev. ed. Portland, OR: Pastoral Press, 1988.

Magesa, Laurenti. "Recognizing the Reality of African Religion in Tanzania." In *Catholic Ethicists on HIV/AIDS Prevention.* Edited by James F. Keenan, assisted by Jon D. Fuller, Lisa Sowle Cahill, and Kevin Kelly, 76–84. New York: Continuum, 2000.

Mahoney, John. "The Making of Moral Theology: A Study of the Roman Catholic Tradition." *The Martin D'Arcy Memorial Lectures 1981–1982.* Oxford: Oxford University Press, 1987.

Marins, J. R., L. F. Jamal, S. Y. Chen, M. B. Barros, E. S. Hudes, A. A. Barbosa, P. Chequer, P. R. Teixeira, and N. Hearst. "Dramatic Improvement in Survival among Adult Brazilian AIDS Patients." *AIDS* 17, no. 11 (2003): 1675–82.

Martin, Emily. *The Woman in the Body: A Cultural Analysis of Reproduction.* Boston: Beacon, 1987.

McAuliffe, Patricia. *Fundamental Ethics: A Liberationist Approach.* Washington, DC: Georgetown University Press, 1993.

McCarthy, Donald G., Ph.D., and Edward J. Bayer, S.T.D. *Handbook on Critical Sexual Issues.* Garden City, NY: Doubleday, 1984.

McDonagh, Enda. "The Reign of God: Signposts for Catholic Moral Theology." In *Catholic Ethicists on HIV/AIDS Prevention.* Edited by James F. Keenan, assisted by Jon D. Fuller, Lisa Sowle Cahill, and Kevin Kelly, 317–23. New York: Continuum, 2000.

———. "Theology in a Time of AIDS." *Irish Theological Quarterly* 60 (1994): 81–99.

McGeary, Johanna, "Death Stalks a Continent." *Time*, 12 February 2001, 42.

———. "Paying for AIDS Cocktails: Who Should Pick Up the Tab for the Third World?" *Time*, 12 February 2001, 54.

McKenny, Gerald P. *To Relieve the Human Condition: Bioethics, Technology, and the Body.* Albany, NY: State University of New York Press, 1997.

Meeks, Wayne A. *The Moral World of the First Christians.* Philadelphia: Westminster Press, 1986.

———, ed. *HarperCollins Study Bible*, New Revised Standard Version. New York: HarperCollins, 1993.

"Merck Leads New Round of AIDS Drug Price Cuts." *Reuters*, 7 March, 2001.

Merson, M. H. *TASO Uganda: The Inside Story.* Kampala, Uganda: Marianum Press, 1995.

"A Message of Hope from the Catholic Bishops to the People of God in South Africa, Botswana and Swaziland." Presented at the Southern African Bishops' Conference, 30 July 2001.

Metz, Johannes Baptist. *Poverty of Spirit.* Translated by John Drury. Paramus, NJ: Newman Press, 1968.

———. *Faith in History and Society: Toward a Practical Fundamental Theology.* Translated by David Smith. New York: Seabury Press, 1980.

———. *The Emergent Church: The Future of Christianity in a Postbourgeois World.* Translated by Peter Mann. New York: Crossroad, 1981.

———. "Communicating a Dangerous Memory." In *Communicating a Dangerous Memory: Soundings in Political Theology.* Edited by Fred Lawrence. Atlanta: Scholars Press, 1987.

———. "With the Eyes of a European Theologian." *Concilium* 6 (1990): 113–19.

———. "God and the Evil of This World: Forgotten, Unforgettable Theodicy." In *The Return of the Plague.* Edited by Jose Oscar Beozzo and Virgilio Elizondo. London: SCM Press, 1997.

———. *A Passion for God: The Mystical-Political Dimension of Christianity.* Edited and translated by J. Matthew Ashley. New York: Paulist Press, 1998.

Ministerio de Salud de Argentina. *Boletin sobre el SIDA en la Argentina.* Ano X, Numero 22. Buenos Aires: Ministerio de Salud, October 2003.

Mofenson, Lunn. "Short-Course Zidovudine for Prevention of Perinatal Infection." *Lancet* 353 (6 March 1999): 766–67.

Moser, Antonio, and Bernardino Leers. *Moral Theology: Dead Ends and Alternatives.* Translated by Paul Burns. Maryknoll, NY: Orbis Books, 1990.

Murphy, Sheila. *A Delicate Dance: Sexuality, Celibacy, and Relationships among Catholic Clergy and Religious.* With an introduction by Donald J. Goergen, O.P. New York: Crossroad, 1992.

Murphy, Timothy F. *Ethics in an Epidemic: AIDS, Morality and Culture.* Berkeley, CA: University of California Press, 1994.

Mushete, A. Ngindu. "An Overview of African Theology." In *Paths of African Theology.* Edited by Rosino Gibellini, 9–26. Maryknoll, NY: Orbis Books, 1994.

Mveng, Engelbert. "Impoverishment and Liberation: A Theological Approach for Africa and the Third World." In *Paths of African Theology.* Edited by Rosino Gibellini, 154–65. Maryknoll, NY: Orbis Books, 1994.

Myers, Bryant L. *Walking with the Poor: Principles and Practices of Transformational Development.* Maryknoll, NY: Orbis Books, 1999.

National Conference of Catholic Bishops (NCCB). *Called to Compassion and Responsibility: A Response to the HIV/AIDS Crisis.* Washington, DC: USCC, November 1989.

———. *Economic Justice for All: Pastoral Letter on Catholic Social Teaching and the U.S. Economy.* Washington, DC: USCC, 1986.

National Institute of Allergy and Infectious Diseases (NIAID). *HIV Infection and AIDS (March 1999),* 1, 4. Available at http://www.aegis.com/topics/basics/whataidsis.html. Internet. Accessed December 1999.

Nelson, Daniel Mark. *The Priority of Prudence.* University Park, PA: Pennsylvania State University Press, 1992.

Nelson, James B. *Embodiment: An Approach to Sexuality and Christian Theology.* Minneapolis, MN: Augsburg Publishing House, 1978.

Nelson, James B., and Sandra P. Longfellow, eds. *Sexuality and the Sacred: Sources for Theological Reflection.* Louisville, KY: Westminster/John Knox Press, 1994.

Nugent, Robert. *Prayer Journey for Persons with AIDS.* Cincinnati, OH: St. Anthony Messenger, 1989.

Nussbaum, Martha C. "Non-Relative Virtues: An Aristotelian Approach." In *Ethical Theory: Character and Virtue.* Midwest Studies in Philosophy 13. Edited by P. French, T. Uehling, and H. Wettstein, 32–53. Notre Dame, IN: University of Notre Dame Press, 1988.

———. *Sex and Social Justice.* New York: Oxford University Press, 1999.

———. *Women and Human Development: The Capabilities Approach.* Cambridge and New York: Cambridge University Press, 2000.

O'Brien, David J., and Thomas A. Shannon, eds. In *Catholic Social Thought: The Documentary Heritage.* Maryknoll, NY: Orbis Books, 1992.

O'Connell, Timothy E. *Making Disciples: A Handbook of Christian Moral Formation.* New York: Crossroad Publishing, 1998.

Oduyoye, Mercy Amba. *Hearing and Knowing: Theological Reflections on Christianity in Africa.* Maryknoll, NY: Orbis Books, 1986.

———. *Who Will Roll the Stone Away? The Ecumenical Decade of the Churches in Solidarity with Women.* Geneva, Switzerland: World Council of Churches, 1990.

———. *Daughters of Anowa: African Women and Patriarchy.* Maryknoll, NY: Orbis Books, 1995.

———. "Feminist Theology in an African Perspective." In *Paths of African Theology.* Edited by Rosino Gibellini, 166–81. Maryknoll, NY: Orbis Books, 1994.

———. "A Coming Home to Myself: The Childless Woman in the West African Space." In *Liberating Eschatology: Essays in Honor of Letty M. Russell.* Edited by Margaret A. Farley and Serene Jones, 105–20. Louisville, KY: Westminster John Knox Press, 1999.

———, ed. "Transforming Power: Women in the Household of God." Proceedings of the Pan African Conference of the Circle of Concerned African Women Theologians, 1997.

Oduyoye, Mercy Amba, and Musimbi R. A. Kanyoro, eds. *The Will to Arise: Women, Tradition, and the Church in Africa.* Maryknoll, NY: Orbis Books, 1992.

O'Keefe, Mark, OSB. *Becoming Good, Becoming Holy: On the Relationship of Christian Ethics and Spirituality.* New York: Paulist Press, 1995.

O'Keefe, Mark. "Liturgical Preaching and the Moral Life of Christians." In *Spirituality and Moral Theology: Essays from a Pastoral Perspective.* Edited by James Keating, 44. New York: Paulist Press, 2000.

Okure, Teresa, SHCJ. "HIV and Women: Gender Issues, Culture and Church." Paper presented at the Consultation on HIV/AIDS, Bertoni Centre, Pretoria, April 2000, 1–13.

Outka, Gene. *Agape: An Ethical Analysis.* New Haven, CT: Yale University Press, 1972.

Overberg, Kenneth R., ed. *AIDS, Ethics and Religion: Embracing a World of Suffering.* Maryknoll, NY: Orbis Books, 1994.

Palmer, C. J., L. Validum, B. Loeffke, H. E. Laubach, C. Mitchell, R. Cummings, and R. R. Cuadrado. "HIV Prevalence in a Gold Mining Camp in the Amazon region, Guyana." *Emerging Infectious Diseases* 8, no. 3 (March 2002). Available at http://www.cdc.gov/ncidod/eid/vol8no3/01-0261.htm.

Parker, Richard G. "Empowerment, Community Mobilization, and Social Change in the Face of HIV/AIDS." Paper presented at the XI International Conference on AIDS, Vancouver, July 1996.

Parsons, Susan Frank. *Feminism and Christian Ethics.* Cambridge and New York: University of Cambridge Press, 1996.

Partners in Health. Brochure. See website at http://www.pih.org/index.html.

Patrick, Anne E. "Ethics and Spirituality: The Social Justice Connection." *The Way* 63, Suppl. (1988): 103–16.

———. *Liberating Conscience: Feminist Explorations in Catholic Moral Theology.* New York: Continuum, 1997.

Peterson, V. Spike, and Anne Sisson Runyan. *Global Gender Issues,* 2nd ed. Boulder, CO: Westview Press, 1999.

Philibert, Paul J. O. P. "Memory." In *The New Dictionary of Catholic Spirituality.* Edited by Michael Downey, 651–53. Collegeville, MN: Liturgical Press, 1993.

Pieper, Josef. *Prudence*. Translated by Richard Winston and Clara Winston. New York: Pantheon Books, 1959.

Pilla, Bishop Anthony M. "Statement on Developing an Approach by the Church to AIDS Education." *Origins* 16 (1987): 692–93.

Piot, Peter. "Preface." In *Report on the Global HIV/AIDS Epidemic, 2002*. Joint United Nations Programme on HIV/AIDS (UNAIDS), 6. Available at http://www.unaids.org/barcelona/presskit/barcelona%20report/preface.html. Internet. Accessed 10 October 2002.

———. "Preface." In *Report on the Global HIV/AIDS Epidemic, 2000*. Joint United Nations Programme on HIV/AIDS (UNAIDS), 1.

———. "Message on the Occasion of World AIDS Day." Available at http://www.unaids.org/html/pub/media/speeches02/SP_Piot_WAD2004_01Dec04_en_pdf. Internet. Accessed 27 December 2004.

Pleins, J. David. "'Why Do You Hide Your Face?' Divine Silence and Speech in the Book of Job." *Interpretation* 48 (July 1994): 229–40.

———. "Suffering and the Christian Tradition." *Yale Journal for Humanities in Medicine*, 4. Available at http://info.med.yale.edu/intmed/hummed/yjhm/spirit/suffering/jkeenanprint.htm. Internet. Accessed 10 September 2003.

Pohl, Christine D. *Making Room: Recovering Hospitality as a Christian Tradition*. Grand Rapids, MI: Eerdmans Publishing, 1999.

Pope John Paul II. *Laborem Exercens (On Human Work)*. Washington, DC: Office of Publishing Services, 1981.

———. "*Sollicitudo Rei Socialis* (On Social Concern)." In *Catholic Social Thought: The Documentary Heritage*. Edited by David J. O'Brien and Thomas A. Shannon, 393–436. Maryknoll, NY: Orbis Books, 1992.

———. *The Theology of the Body: Human Love in the Divine* Plan. Boston, MA: Pauline Books, 1997.

Pope Paul VI. *Populorum Progressio* (1967).

———. "Encyclical Letter on the Regulation of Births." *Humanae Vitae*, 25 July 1968. In *Vatican Council II: More Postconciliar Documents*, English ed. Edited by Austin Flannery. Grand Rapids, MI: Eerdmans, 1982.

Pope, Stephen. "Expressive Individualism and True Self-Love: A Thomistic Perspective." *Journal of Religion* 71.3 (1991): 384–99.

———. *The Evolution of Altruism and the Ordering of Love*. Washington, DC: Georgetown University Press, 1994.

———, ed. *The Ethics of Aquinas*. Washington, DC: Georgetown University Press, 2002.

Porter, Jean. "Virtue Ethics and Its Significance for Spirituality." *The Way* 88, Suppl. (Spring 1997): 26–35.

———. *The Recovery of Virtue: The Relevance of Aquinas for Christian Ethics*. Louisville, KY: Westminster/John Knox Press, 1990.

———. "The Virtue of Justice (IIa IIae, qq. 58–122)." In *The Ethics of Aquinas*. Edited by Stephen J. Pope, 272–86. Washington, DC: Georgetown University Press, 2002.

"Prohibition and Taste: The Bipolarity in Christian Ethics." *Ethical Perspectives* 1, no. 3 (September 1994): 130–44.

Rahner, Karl, and Johann Baptist Metz. *The Courage to Pray*. Translated by Sarah O'Brien Twohig. New York: Crossroad, 1981.

Rausch, Thomas P. "Discipleship." In *The New Dictionary of Catholic Spirituality*. Edited by Michael Downey, 281–84. Collegeville, MN: Liturgical Press, 1993.

Rolheiser, Ronald. *The Holy Longing: The Search for a Christian Spirituality*. New York: Doubleday, 1999.

Rosenberg, Tina. "How to Solve the World's AIDS Crisis." *New York Times Magazine*, 28 January 2001, 26.

———. "Look at Brazil." *New York Times Magazine*, 28 January 2001, 26.

Rosenthal, Elisabeth. "China Raises Estimates of H.I.V.-AIDS Cases to 1 Million." *New York Times*, 6 September 2002.

———. "AIDS Scourge in Rural China Leaves Village of Orphans." *New York Times*, 25 October 2002.

Rotter, Hans. "AIDS: Some Theological and Pastoral Considerations." *Theology Digest* 39 (1992): 235–39.

Ruffing, Janet K. "Anthropology, Theological." In *The New Dictionary of Catholic Spirituality*. Edited by Michael Downey, 47–50. Collegeville, MN: Liturgical Press, 1993.

Russell, Letty M. "Liberation Theology in a Feminist Perspective." In *Liberation, Revolution, and Freedom: Theological Perspectives. Proceedings of the College Theology Society*. Edited by Thomas M. McFadden, 88–107. New York: Crossroad, 1975.

Sadik, Nafis. "Gender Dimensions of HIV/AIDS: A Key Challenge to Rural Development." United Nations, New York, 30 April 2004, 6. Available at http://www.un.org/esa/coordination/ecosoc/hl2003/RT2%20Sadik.pdf. Internet. Accessed 30 June 2004.

Salzman, Todd A., ed. *Method and Catholic Moral Theology: The Ongoing Reconstruction*. Omaha, NE: Creighton University Press, 1999.

Schaeffer, Pamela. "Condoms Tolerated to Avoid AIDS, French Bishops Say." *National Catholic Reporter*. 23 February 1996, 9.

Schillebeeckx, Edward. *Christ, the Sacrament of the Encounter with God*. New York: Sheed & Ward, 1963.

———. *Jesus: An Experiment in Christology*. Translated by Hubert Hoskins. New York: Seabury, 1979.

———. *Christ: The Experience of Jesus as Lord*. Translated by John Bowden. New York: Crossroad, 1981.

Schneiders, Sandra M. "Theology and Spirituality: Strangers, Rivals, or Partners?" *Horizons* 13 (Fall 1986): 253–74.

———. "Spirituality in the Academy." *Theological Studies* 50, no. 4 (1989): 676–97.

———. "Spirituality as an Academic Discipline: Reflections from Experience." *In Broken and Whole: Essays on Religion and the Body*. Edited by Maureen A. Tilley and Susan A. Ross. Lanham, MD: University Press of America, 1993.

———. *The Revelatory Text: Interpreting the New Testament as Sacred Scripture*, 2nd ed. Collegeville, MN: Liturgical Press, 1999.

———. "With Oil in Their Lamps: Faith, Feminism, and the Future." *2000 Madeleva Lecture in Spirituality*. New York: Paulist Press, 2000.

Schoofs, Mark, and Michael Waldholz. "Price War Breaks Out Over AIDS Drugs in Africa as Generics Present Challenge." *Wall Street Journal*, 7 March 2001.

Schreiter, Robert J., CPPS. *The Ministry of Reconciliation: Spirituality and Strategies*. Maryknoll, NY: Orbis Books, 1998.

Schuster, Ekkehard, and Reinhold Boschert-Kimmig. *Hope Against Hope: Johann Baptist Metz and Elie Wiesel Speak Out on the Holocaust.* Translated by J. Matthew Ashley. New York: Paulist, 1999.

Second Vatican Council. "Gaudium et Spes." *Pastoral Constitution on the Church in the Modern World.* 1965.

Sellers, Deborah E., Sarah A. McGraw, and John B. McKinlay. "Does the Promotion and Distribution of Condoms Increase Teen Sexual Activity? Evidence from an HIV Prevention Program for Latino Youth." *American Journal of Public Health* 84 (December 1994): 1952–59.

Sen, Amartya. *Development as Freedom.* New York: Alfred A. Knopf, 1999.

Sheldrake, Philip. *Spirituality and Theology: Christian Living and the Doctrine of God.* Maryknoll, NY: Orbis Books, 1998.

Shengli, C., Z. Shikun, and S. B. Westley. "HIV/AIDS Awareness Is Improving in China." *Asia-Pacific Population & Policy* 69 (2004): 1-5.

Simon, Yves R. *The Definition of Moral Virtue.* Edited by Vukan Kuic, 96–98. New York: Fordham University Press, 1986.

Sobrino, Jon. *Jesus in Latin America.* Maryknoll, NY: Orbis Books, 1987.

———. "Bearing with One Another in Faith." In *Theology of Christian Solidarity.* Edited by Jon Sobrino and Juan Hernández Pico. Translated by Phillip Berryman, 1–44. Maryknoll, NY: Orbis Books, 1985.

———. *Spirituality of Liberation: Toward Political Holiness.* Translated by Robert R. Barr. Maryknoll, NY: Orbis Books, 1988.

———. *The Principle of Mercy: Taking the Crucified People from the Cross.* Maryknoll, NY: Orbis Books, 1994.

Sobrino, Jon, SJ, and Juan Hernández Pico, SJ. *Theology of Christian Solidarity.* Translated by Phillip Berryman. Maryknoll, NY: Orbis Books, 1982.

Soelle, Dorothee. *Suffering.* Translated by Everett R. Kalin. Philadelphia: Fortress Press, 1975.

"South African Bishops to Discuss AIDS, Condom Use." *Catholic News Service,* 11 July 2001.

Spohn, William C. "The Return of Virtue Ethics." *Theological Studies* 53 (1992): 60–75.

———. *Go and Do Likewise: Jesus and Ethics.* New York: Continuum, 2000.

St. John, M. A. et al. "Efficacy of Nevirapine Administration on Mother-to-Child Transmission of HIV Using a Modified HIVNET 012 Regimen." *West Indian Medical Journal* 51, Suppl. 3 (2003): 1–87.

Steinhauer, Jennifer. "Undeterred by a Monster: Secrecy and Stigma Keep AIDS Risk High for Gay Black Men." *New York Times,* 11 February 2001, NE31.

Stiltner, Brian. *Religion and the Common Good: Catholic Contributions to Building Community in a Liberal Society.* Lanham, MD: Rowman & Littlefield Publishers, 1999.

"Study in 6 Cities Finds HIV in 30% of Young Black Gays." *New York Times,* 6 February 2001.

Synod of Bishops. "Justice in the World 1971." In *Catholic Social Thought: The Documentary Heritage.* Edited by David J. O'Brien and Thomas A. Shannon, 287–300. Maryknoll, NY: Orbis Books, 1992.

Theunissen, Michael. *The Other: Studies in the Social Ontology of Husserl, Heidegger, Sartre, and Buber.* Translated by C. Macann. Cambridge: MIT Press, 1984.

Tillmann, Fritz. *The Master Calls: A Handbook of Christian Living*. Baltimore: Helicon Press, 1960.

Toombs, S. Kay. "Illness and the Paradigm of Lived Body." *Theoretical Medicine* 9 (1988): 201–26.

Townes, Emilie M. *Breaking the Fine Rain of Death: African American Health Issues and a Womanist Ethic of Care*. New York: Continuum, 1998.

Tracy, David. *The Analogical Imagination: Christian Theology and the Culture of Pluralism*. New York: Crossroad, 1981.

United Nations General Assembly Special Session on HIV/AIDS, June 2001, New York, para. 55, 62.

United States Catholic Council of Bishops (USCCB). *Human Sexuality: A Catholic Perspective for Education and Lifelong Learning*. Washington, DC: USCC, 1997.

———. *The Many Faces of AIDS: A Gospel Response: A Statement of the Administrative Board*. Washington, DC: USCC, 1987.

United States Census Bureau. *Annual Estimates of the Population by Sex, Race and Hispanic or Latino Origin for the United States: April 1, 2000 to July 1, 2003*. Washington, 2004.

———. *Poverty Status of the Population in 1999 by Age, Sex, Race and Hispanic Origin*. Washington, 2000.

United States Centers for Disease Control and Prevention. *HIV/AIDS Surveillance Report* 10, no. 2 (1998): 1–43.

———. *HIV/AIDS Surveillance Report* 15 (2004). CDC, Presentation by Dr. Harold Jaffe, "HIV/AIDS in America Today," National HIV Prevention Conference, 2003. Cited in Henry J. Kaiser Family Foundation, "The HIV/AIDS Epidemic in the United States," December 2004. *HIV/AIDS Policy Fact Sheet*. Available at http://www.kff.org. Internet. Accessed 12 December 2004.

———. *HIV/AIDS Among African-Americans*, 2003. Available at http://www.cdc.gov/hiv/pubs/facts/afam.htm. Internet. Accessed 27 December 2004.

———. *HIV/AIDS Among African-Americans*. Fact Sheet. Washington, DC: U.S. Centers for Disease Control and Prevention. Available at http://www.cdc.gov/hiv/pubs/facts/afam.htm. Internet. Accessed 16 September 2004.

Vacek, Edward Collins, SJ. *Love, Human and Divine: The Heart of Christian Ethics*. Washington, DC: Georgetown University Press, 1994.

Vatican Council II: The Conciliar and Post Conciliar Documents, new rev. ed. Edited by Austin Flannery. Vatican Collection, Vol. 1. Grand Rapids, MI: Eerdmans Publishing Co., 1992.

Vatican Council II. *Gaudium et Spes*. In *Catholic Social Thought: The Documentary Heritage*. Edited by David J. O'Brien and Thomas A. Shannon, 164–237. Maryknoll, NY: Orbis Books, 1992.

"Vienna Archbishop Says Condoms Morally Acceptable to Fight AIDS." *Catholic News Service*, 3 April 1996.

Vitillo, Robert. "HIV/AIDS Prevention Education: A Special Concern for the Church." Presentation for discussion at Caritas Internationalis, CAFOD Theological Consultation on HIV/AIDS, Pretoria, South Africa, 14 April 1998.

Waliggo, John Mary. "A Woman Confronts Social Stigma in Uganda." In *Catholic Ethicists on HIV/AIDS Prevention*. Edited by James F. Keenan, assisted by Jon D. Fuller, Lisa Sowle Cahill, and Kevin Kelly, 48–56. New York: Continuum, 2000. Available at www.hdnet.org/Stigma/Meeting%20Agenda%20and%20presentations/Keynote%20address.htm.

Weeks, Jeffrey. *Invented Moralities: Sexual Values in an Age of Uncertainty*. New York: Columbia University Press, 1995.

Weil, Simone. *Waiting for God*. Translated by Emma Craufurd. New York: Harper & Row, 1973.

Whitney, Craig. "French Bishop Supports Some Use of Condoms to Prevent AIDS." *New York Times*, 13 February 1996, 5.

"Wife-beating in Zambia a 'Natural Consequence.'" *Mail & Guardian Online*, 17 September 2004. Available at http://www.mg.co.za/Content/13.asp?ao=24385. Internet. Accessed 17 September 2004.

Williams, Bernard. "Justice as a Virtue." In *Essays on Aristotle's Ethics*. Edited by Amerial Oksenberg Rorty, 189–99. Berkeley, CA: University of California Press, 1980.

Woodill, William Joseph. *The Fellowship of Life: Virtue Ethics and Orthodox Christianity*. Washington, DC: Georgetown University Press, 1998.

World Health Organization. *World Health Report, 1999*.

———. "Key Facts from the World Health Report 2004." *The World Health Report 2004: Changing History*. May 2004.

Wyschogrod, Edith. *Saints and Postmodernism*. Chicago: University of Chicago Press, 1990.

Yearley, Lee H. "Recent Work on Virtue." *Religious Studies Review* 16 (1990): 2.

Zacharias, Ronaldo, SDB. "Virtue Ethics as the Framework for Catholic Sexual Education: Towards the Integration between Being and Acting in Sexual Education." STD dissertation, Weston Jesuit School of Theology, 2002.

Zambia Demographic Health Survey, 2001–2002. Calverton, MD: Central Statistics Office and Macro International Inc. February 2003.

Index